THE
DOCTOR'S
SORE FOOT
BOOK

THE DOCTOR'S SORE FOOT BOOK

Daniel M. McGann, DPM,
and L. R. Robinson
Drawings by Eric Miller

William Morrow and Company, Inc.
New York

Copyright © 1991 by Daniel M. McGann, D P M, and L. R. Robinson

It is the policy of William Morrow and Company, Inc., and its imprints and affiliates, recognizing the importance of preserving what has been written, to print the books we publish on acid-free paper, and we exert our best efforts to that end.

Library of Congress Cataloging-in-Publication Data

McGann, Daniel M.
    The doctor's sore foot book / Daniel M. McGann and L. R. Robinson : drawings by Eric Miller.
        p.   cm.
    Includes bibliographical references and index.
    ISBN 0-688-09117-2
    1. Foot—Care and hygiene.   2. Foot—Diseases.   I. Robinson, L. R. II. Title.
    RD563.M38   1991
    617.5'85—dc20   90-27307
                                                                                   CIP

Printed in the United States of America

First Edition

1 2 3 4 5 6 7 8 9 10

BOOK DESIGN BY ARLENE GOLDBERG

For
Adele, Leslie, and David

Contents

Introduction
Your Feet—Where They Are
And What They Are

Feet. Save for a very few rather, um, special people, feet don't bring forth images of true love, unimaginable wealth, or long-sought fame. Truth to tell, you hardly ever think about feet when they're working the way they're supposed to.

But when they're not, it can be murder. "My feet are killing me": That statement echoes through millions of homes throughout the world every day. In the United States the leading cause of rejection for military service during World War II was foot disability. The Bible chronicles the great accomplishments of King Asa, David's son, but "nevertheless in the time of his old age he was diseased in his feet." (I Kings 15:23).

Bad feet are suffered alone. That's why hypochondriacs rarely have bad feet as their symptom of choice. But those of you who have bad feet don't have the luxury of choice. It does you no good to pretend you suffer from a spastic colon or migraines or whatever. It really *is* your feet that hurt.

But if you don't have the choice of symptom, at least you do have the option of making your bad feet good. You may not make your feet the envy of all your friends, but you can eradicate the pain that makes you think about your feet so much of the time. The ways in which you can do this is the subject of this book.

It might be better if we had wheels to carry us the 250,000 miles we will ultimately travel, but we don't. And a lot of localized troubles in adult life are caused by improper shoes and faulty muscular development. Many systemic diseases can cause serious foot problems as well.

A cleverly designed wheel would avoid the main source of most foot problems: the enormous pressure of the weight we put on our feet. This pressure varies from person to person. It's said that Orson Welles asked of his feet a resistance to pressure that no manmade machine was capable of until 1967. Twiggy, on the other hand, practically had to be nailed down to keep from floating away. Most of us fall between these two extremes, but close enough to Mighty Orson to make the weight our feet must handle a potential source of all sorts of trouble.

As a species that walks upright we are mere babes. As babies we haltingly, and not always successfully, rise from all fours to a walking position. Perhaps future species will adapt completely to bipedal movement, but we have not. As a result we pay for the obvious advantages with feet that bear the brunt of incompletely successful evolution.

Feets of Strength?

When you consider what your feet have to do, it's easy to see why they develop so many problems. An average man of average weight (165 to 170 pounds) walks seven and one-half miles on an average day. This requires *each* foot to carry more than five hundred tons a day, and we're not even talking about postmen and meter inspectors. The demands made on their feet by women's lighter bodies are, of course, somewhat less, but women have cleverly gained equality here by wearing shoes that might as well have been designed by the most greedy and immoral manufacturer of worthless foot remedies. Recent studies have revealed that high heels put 76 percent more pressure on the balls of your feet than going barefoot. Very high heels shorten the normal gait stride, which requires more steps to cover a given distance.

Have you ever seen a small child run happily over stones that would cause excruciating pain were you to follow? Small children are immune to many of the foot problems that afflict adults because the weight of the child's body (relative to the ability of the foot to resist) is much less.

When children do have foot problems, it is often not nature that is at fault. Human ingenuity being what it is, we have managed to mess up the feet of many children whose feet would have been fine were it not for our attempts to make them fine. Perhaps the chief contributing factor is overanxious parents' attempts to teach their toddlers to walk too early. The average child begins to walk in his fourteenth month; left alone by his folks, he would not attempt to walk this early. He would hold off until the musculature of his feet had developed sufficiently to balance the human tendency for the ankle to "roll in." Likewise he would, if he could talk, tell his parents that there is no point—indeed that it is harmful—to wear shoes until he is walking full-time.

As if premature attempts to get the child to walk were not damaging enough, many parents fail to realize that the softness of the child's foot renders it extremely vulnerable to deformation by pressure. Tight shoes and other foot coverings are the primary cause of such pressure.

Why are a baby's feet so important? To begin with, his feet must last a lifetime. Remember, a child has those 250,000 miles ahead of him. He can make this journey on strong, healthy feet or join the ranks of thousands moaning every step of the way. When your feet hurt, you hurt all over! Any adult with bad feet will tell you that is absolutely true.

The baby's foot grows at an enormous rate. By the age of one it is half its eventual adult length. Not just shoes but socks, crib slippers, "footies," and even bed clothing can constrict this growth and guarantee later problems.

It would be bad enough if our well-meant, but harmful, attempts damaged only the child's *foot*. But the reality is much worse: Just as problems far removed from the feet can cause foot problems, so can foot problems cause problems far removed from the feet. Many an adult's bad posture and back pain can be traced to poor foot practices at an early age.

Moreover it is far from unreasonable to suggest that, when children do have bad feet, the effects can express themselves even in personality difficulties in adulthood. Consider the child who, as a result of one of a number of possible foot problems, walks in an awkward, unbecoming manner and has a shuffling gait and bad posture. Every podiatrist has seen a number of such children. They often encounter unfriendliness, and even jibes, from their classmates, and respond by developing a shyness and introversion that can, in the worst cases, last a lifetime.

To the extent that the young do escape foot problems, the old suffer from them. Indeed foot problems develop almost linearly with age: The older you get, the more likely you are to have problems with your feet. However, younger adults are not let off easy. Because they are more likely to engage in activities that are unusually hard on the feet, twenty- and thirty-year-olds are far from unacquainted with the foot doctor's trade.

In short, at one time or another 85 percent of all Americans have foot problems serious enough to require professional attention. In nursing homes this figure rises to near 100 percent!

Uninformed Self-Medication: Prescription for Foot Disorders

Most people who have bad feet, however, never go to the foot doctor. They often raise woefully wrong self-medication to the level of high art and prescribe for themselves "solutions" that are precisely the opposite of what they should be doing to solve their problems.

The primary reason why so many people go so wrong is that the causes of foot problems are rarely obvious. The exquisite way in which the bones and other materials of the foot carry the body permits a low tolerance for error or misalignment. Thus a slight imbalance of a body part far away from the foot can manifest itself in a deformation of the foot. Common sense is rarely much of a help here. You have to know what you are doing, and when it comes to feet, most people don't.

So, when most people hobble into their local drugstores to buy something to fix their ailing feet, or at least to dull the pain, they buy the very thing that is most likely to make matters worse and to increase the pain. And even when such seat-of-the-pants remedies don't actually make things worse, they delay the time before proper procedures are instituted, giving the malady more time to develop.

The Social Cost of Bad Feet

The problem extends far beyond the individual. Indeed it is not exaggeration to say that the bad feet of individuals results in a major problem for all of society. When your feet hurt so badly that you can't go to work, the company you work for is less productive that day. When a million people take off a million days from work, we have a major social problem. And every year bad feet cause hundreds of thousands of people to take off many more than one day from work.

Add into this the fact that over a quarter of all household accidents injure feet. (Remember the last time you smacked your toe into the bedpost?) Self-inflicted mismedication after such accidents swells the eventual number of absent workers and therefore the cost of producing goods.

Perhaps the most tragic of the results of unsupervised self-medication occur when the foot is not the source of the malady but its symptom. Here enormous medical costs, for the individual and for society, can result when a serious disease is self-diagnosed as a minor foot problem. Dry skin, brittle nails, insensitivity, discoloration, and a host of other symptoms are usually minor, but they can also be symptoms of diabetes, vascular problems, and a number of circulatory disorders. In other cases diseases seemingly unrelated to feet get their start when feet go bad: arthritic knees, leg deformations, and a wide range of lower-back problems could be avoided if everyone attended to his feet at the appropriate time.

Historic Feets

At least we have the satisfaction of knowing that we did not invent the practices that do so much to destroy what nature attempts to create. While we have extended the problem by creating an economic system that brings shoes to the formerly shoeless, and healthy-footed, strata of society, the upper classes of virtually every society on which we have evidence have done their damnedest to destroy their very means of locomotion.

It is assumed that the peoples of prehistory wore thonged animal hides that offered no more support than did the moccasins of the first American Indians. Such footwear probably did little harm, certainly far less than the sandals that graced the feet of Egyptian ladies. On the next trip to your local museum take a look at these torture racks bejeweled with pointed doodads that look more like what one would wish on an enemy than on the leading ladies of one's own nation. It is one of those small but satisfying ironies that the slaves of these aristocrats had unshod, and very healthy, feet.

You no doubt have heard of Achilles, whose mom tried to protect him against all dangers by dipping him in a tub. Alas, Mom forgot to dip the heel she held when she dipped Achilles. Needless to say, Achilles got it right in the you-know-where when he grew up to be a warrior.

Like all myths, this one has a moral: In protecting one part you may make another one vulnerable. We shall see how an attempt to reduce pressure on, say, the ball of the foot can introduce problems to the instep that had previously been the envy of instep aficionados (an admittedly small but fervent group).

The Romans started the fad of owning more than one pair of shoes (not a bad idea), but none of them were much worth owning: thong-type sandals that were hard and lent no support at all.

Foot trouble is one area where women have men beat, hands down. Thanks to some of the truly absurd footwear fashions of the past and present (and future, too, I'm sure), women leave men at the starting gate.

The people of ancient Turkey wore a wooden sole a foot off the ground, supported by four sticks. One wonders what they were afraid of stepping in. Not to be outdone by the East, English gentlemen of the early Middle Ages wore shoes with toes so long they had to be held up with chains attached to the knees. A century later Venetian ladies wore shoes an inch higher than those of the Turks.

For a thousand years, well into the twentieth century, Chinese women practiced the custom of foot binding that quite literally left them crippled for life. Beginning at about age five for a period of three-plus years, a girl's feet were bound and strapped daily until the desired length of three and one-half to four inches was reached but not exceeded. Outer toes were flexed upon the sole and metatarsals squeezed together. Later the entire forefoot was manipulated into a plantar flexed position. The cone-shaped foot was placed into smaller and smaller shoes in order to maintain the desired length. The resulting deformity severely limited the ability to walk, to the point where women had to be squired around town in sedan chairs. What is truly fascinating is that this horribly deformed foot was considered the most intimate part of a woman's body and an overwhelmingly erotic source of sexual arousal for men. The fondling of feet was an important part of foreplay. In late nineteenth-century China photos of unbound feet were considered pornographic. And you think whips and chains are bad!

Thank goodness American know-how finally came to the rescue, right? Well, not exactly. Seems that early American shoemakers didn't find it necessary to distinguish left shoes from right. Now, you might suppose this means that early American shoemakers believed people had identical right and left feet, but that was obviously not the case. Manufacturers simply found it was cheaper to make both shoes the same. And colonial foot doctors did *very* well indeed.

The human foot has been called a mirror of health, and it is true that many of the early signs of serious systemic diseases are first manifested in the foot.

The foot is a very sophisticated structure, and before any discussion of its many maladies can be undertaken, a basic understanding of its function and anatomy are necessary. This will be presented in considerable detail in the chapter on anatomy and terminology.

For now, it is important to remember that there are twenty-eight bones in the human foot. Our big toes have two bones each, the distal and proximal phalanx. The smaller toes, the second through the pinkie, all have three bones, the distal, middle, and proximal phalanx. There are five metatarsals, three cuneiform bones, one cuboid, one talus, and one calcaneous (heel) bone. The toes (phalanges) and the metatarsals make up the forefoot. The cuneiform, cuboid, talus, and calcaneous make up the rearfoot. There are also two small, round bones under the first metatarsal near the big toe joint called the sesamoid bones. The inside of the foot (arch side) is called the medial side and the outside of the foot is called the lateral side.

There are six principal ligaments of the foot and ankle. There is a thick, fibrous band of tissue on the bottom of the foot called the plantar fascia that runs longitudinally from the heel to the toes. It acts as a bowstring of the longitudinal arch, aids in propulsion, and supports all structures on the bottom of the foot, which is called the plantar surface.

There is only one dorsal (top) muscle of the foot. The muscles on the plantar (bottom) surface, a total of fifteen, are arranged in four layers from superficial to deep. The layers do not have specific names.

There is a complicated system of arteries and veins, and an equally complicated nervous system. All of these structures can be easily located on the drawings throughout the book.

Even this brief description of the anatomy of the foot can give you an idea of the many structures within the foot that can become diseased, injured, or disfunctional.

The function of the human foot is also complicated. The outer part of the foot is specialized for static weight transmission while the inner part, which is elastic and mobile, is specialized for propulsion. By lying flat on the ground the outer border of the foot forms a buttress for stability and balance. The inner portion is essentially a lever.

The foot performs both static and kinetic functions. Its static function is to support the body. Its kinetic function is to provide leverage for propulsion. The foot acts as a shock absorber on impact and when the body is in motion. It propels the body in walking, climbing, descending, jumping, and dancing. The foot is really a transmitting mechanism to a supporting structure rather than a supporting structure in itself. The basic support is the surface upon which we stand or walk. The pressure felt on the foot while standing or in motion is not exerted by the body's weight but provided by the resistance of the ground. Different supporting structures exert different resistance to the feet. A cork floor or soft ground, having greater resilience than a concrete floor, can exert displacement pressure over a larger area of the foot. Feet that must perform their functions on a hard surface are taxed beyond the intention of functioning on a yielding, supporting surface. Keep in mind those quarter of a million miles we have to cover in our lifetimes.

To understand almost all medical problems, it is necessary to have at least some background information: a pattern, a map, anything that will point the reader in the right direction. For the reader's convenience, this book is divided into two general sec-

tions. Common foot types, tips on foot care, and activities associated with foot problems are presented first. The nuts and bolts
come later in the nature of common foot problems involving specific anatomical structures. Because of the technical nature of some
of this later material it is presented as a reference so that the reader
can more easily access information relating to his or her specific
foot problem. Many of the topics in the beginning of the book will
lay the necessary foundation in order to understand sometimes
complicated concepts later on. As much of the medical mumbo
jumbo as possible has been eliminated. When unfamiliar terms are
used, they are defined in the simplest manner possible. The point
of the whole exercise is to enable the reader to know what he or she
can do to help their painful feet and when to consult a professional.
There are many things you can do to help yourself, and the knowledge within these pages can be the first step toward healthy,
happy, properly functioning feet.

Without question the poor foot is the most neglected part of our
bodies. In nearly thirty years of private practice I have heard every
conceivable question concerning feet. They are all answered in this
book.

Part One

Long Ago and Far Away: Bipedalism and the Evolution of the Foot

On November 30, 1974, Donald Johanson, a paleoanthropologist, found the most complete fossilized skeleton of a single individual that walked the earth erect some 3.5 million years ago. This discovery, made at a place called Hadar in Ethiopia, demonstrated that hominids (near-men) were bipedal approximately one million years earlier than previously thought. The area at Hadar, which is a wasteland of rock, gravel, and sand, is rich in fossils. The temperature can reach over 100 degrees Fahrenheit and it rarely rains there, but when it does, it comes in downpours, and since the local soil is bare of vegetation, it cannot hold the water. The rushing water cuts through the sides of gullies and exposes more fossils. It is because of these changing climatic conditions that important specimens are missed by field expeditions. Either fossils haven't been exposed or good specimens have been washed away. Timing and luck have a lot to do with major finds. The significance of this find lies in the fact that all the bones are from a single individual. No such skeleton had ever been found.

This skeleton came to be known as Lucy (after the Beatles' song): a tiny little thing some three and one-half feet high with a pelvis and leg bones almost identical in function with those of modern man (Homo sapiens). Technically she is from the species *Australopithecus afarensis*.

A second discovery made, at Laetoli, not far from Olduvai Gorge in Tanzania, by members of Mary Leakey's field team, was of equal importance. Bored team members would sometimes amuse themselves by throwing dried elephant dung at one another, a sport of limited participation unless one spends a lot of time at paleontological digs. While dodging a particularly well-aimed shot, Andrew Hill noticed some odd indentations in exposed layers of ash in an ancient streambed. When fully excavated a year later in 1977, fifty footprints covering a distance of seventy-seven feet were revealed. This showed our ancestors walking erect just as we do now some 3.7 million years ago.

The making and preservation of these remarkable footprints is a truly fascinating story. A complicated series of events took place in order for the footprints to survive the millennia.

Laetoli is close to an extinct volcano, Sadiman, that was active four million years ago. Every now and then it would toss out a cloud of carbonite ash (very much like fine beach sand) over the surrounding area, which reached a thickness of about a half inch. Rain rendered the ash into a cementlike layer, which captured clear impressions of every insect or animal walking through the area. The hot sun following the rain quickly dried the ash layer, thus preserving any indentations. Then, before a new rain, good old Sadiman spat out another cloud of ash that covered and sealed the footprints. This pattern of eruptions and hardening of the subsequent layers went on for about a month, producing a protective layer of about eight inches in thickness. Ultimately erosion exposed the prints to our dung dodger. It is amazing how the random events of ash and rain and passing hominids were linked together to leave this important record of modern man's ancestral wanderings.

Why bipedalism? Why bother walking upright? The answer to these questions is considerably more involved than one might suspect. Many factors come into play. Many of the logical arguments are thought to be wrong by locomotion experts. Man's ancestors left the canopy forest, moved out on the savanna, and stood up in order to see over the tall grass. Perfectly logical. Incorrect. Hominids were using bipedal locomotion in the forest long before venturing out on the savanna. They were already bipeds.

Man stood up to free up his hands so he could use tools and weapons. Great idea. Wrong. Early man was walking a million years before he began using tools.

To begin to understand bipedalism, you must examine legs and the quadrupeds first.

The legs of the earliest walking vertebrates go straight out from the sides of their bodies. Alligators that survive today are good examples of this. Later mammals developed legs that stick down instead of going out to the sides. A big improvement on the earlier reptile model. Watch a cheetah run sometime. It is the most highly developed quadrupedal running machine alive. Why bother with bipedal gait if this kind of efficiency is achievable? Because man's ancestors evolved in the trees, and prehensile digits on forepaws were necessary to make a living aloft. Ultimately the primate hand appeared well adapted to climbing. Monkeys developed a primate hand and a primate foot with a flat sole and prehensile digits, and remained quadrupedal. Apes, on the other hand, are designed more for swinging instead of walking along branches.

The gorilla is the one ape that has returned to the ground almost completely and is a true knuckle walker.

Bipedalism frees the forelimbs from gait participation. This fact alone gives significant advantage to sit-and-wait predators. These creatures hunt from a stationary position, and the bipedal hunting posture would have allowed for forward movement during an attack.

In order for evolutionary change to occur, a behavior alteration must be rewarded immediately and be efficient. Nonhuman primates, when they stand erect, must do so in a flexed, bent-hip, bent-knee position. This is very inefficient and leads to early fatigue. Because of this inefficiency forelimbs were used for suspending part of the body weight from overhead points of support, which can be found only in arboreal habitats. This strongly suggests that the first attempts at bipedalism took place in the densely thick canopy of the rain forest several hundred feet off the ground. The rain forest of ancient times provided a rich canopy that could support many life-forms, including carnivorous mammalian predators that hunted there. The demands of this type of hunting style could have provided the selection pressure for the evolution of uprightness.

Members of the cat family, quadrupeds, rely on locomotion and strike while moving. Conversely slow-moving sit-and-wait primitive primates would wait for prey to move into their strike zone. This type of behavior is very restrictive in that one could only capture prey that was within reach of forelimbs, and the range of prey would be limited to those with very low mental powers, such as insects. Mammals anticipate danger and are unlikely to move knowingly into a capture space of a sit-and-wait predator. Because of this our primitive ancestors had to learn to conceal themselves and to hunt from ambush. The dense vegetation of the forest canopy provided the perfect environment for an ambush. This strategy presented new problems, as ambush hunting requires the ability to move forward during the attack to cover the distance to the prey from the hiding place. A slow-moving quadruped that needs its forelimbs for capture cannot combine the attack with purposeful forward movement. Bipedalism frees locomotion from its dependence on forelimb participation. As simple a forward movement as a bipedal lunge sufficient to cover the distance to the prey was all that was necessary for a successful kill. Unfortunately a lot of standing and waiting was required between successful attacks. This demanded the evolution of a musculoskeletal apparatus that permitted the fully extended stance. The weight-bearing system had to be efficient to enable uprightness for long periods of time without excessive energy expenditure. Because of the redesign of the musculo-skeletal structure, early primates were not only able to hunt more efficiently, they were able to travel in the upright position as well.

There are compelling arguments that hominids learned to walk bipedally for sexual and social reasons as well. The giant forests of the time were shrinking significantly and were beginning to get overcrowded. Hominids were breeding successfully, and hands could be put to good use carrying children and food. It was probably the socially and sexually successful ape who became a biped and because of this bipedalism was able to propagate more easily. Somewhere along the line the apelike prehensile foot evolved into the manlike foot.

Our friend Lucy, and other beings from the *Australopithecus afarensis* group, had feet that were functionally the same as those of modern man. Unfortunately no ancestral foot that predates this period exists. The chimpanzee has the nearest model and it is very similar to the gorilla foot.

The foot had to evolve from a partially grasping member into one that can walk. For efficient walking it must act as a platform and provide push-off in stride. The ability to grasp is no longer an important function, so the first evolutionary change would probably have been associated with the big toe. If you picture a chimp's foot, you will note that the big toe is short and sticks out to the side like a thumb. Therefore the first toe would have to be lengthened, made parallel with the lesser toes, and rotated to face downward toward the ground.

Hominids like Lucy had arched phalanges that were considerably longer than the toe bones of man today. Her toes looked very much like fingers. The bones were arched just like bridges to make them stronger and better able to withstand the pull of some very powerful muscles. Apparently some of her time was spent in trees, perhaps sleeping and hiding, which suggests erect quadrupedalism. The entire skeleton gives evidence of extreme ruggedness and strength. They were tough little customers.

There is an interesting theory that the *afarensis* foot was one in transition. The metatarsal joints of a human foot are wide on top and narrow on the bottom. Chimp feet demonstrate the opposite, while the *afarensis* foot shows something in between.

Aside from the changes in the toes, the human foot differs from other models in that it has a medial longitudinal arch. The arch is formed by the shape of the large bones behind the metatarsals (the tarsal bones) and held in place by a thick, fibrous band on the bottom of the foot, called the plantar fascia, and other plantar ligaments. An ape foot is extremely flexible and has no arch. The plantar fascia in the ape foot is poorly developed, as is its heel bone. The human heel bone from behind is on a considerable angle upward and forward to help form the medial longitudinal arch.

Fossil evidence of a foot closely resembling that of modern man's was discovered by Louis Leakey at Olduvai Gorge in Tanzania. This foot is from the species *Australopithecus habilis* (also known as *Homo habilis*), which is dated at about 1.75 million years before the present day. This individual is almost two million years younger than Lucy. The changes that occurred were basically refinements to increase the efficiency of bipedal gait. Although the specimen lacks the back portion of the heel, and the metatarsal heads and toes, it has many characteristics of the human foot. The first metatarsal is clearly in a parallel position to the other metatarsals, essential for efficient bipedal locomotion. It is robust, as is the fifth metatarsal, which indicates weight bearing similar to modern man. The arch is well developed, and there is evidence of well-developed attachment sites from ligamentous structures that maintain the integrity of the medial longitudinal arch.

Homo erectus lived during a period from 1.5 million to 400,000 years ago. There are many fossils from this group, but oddly enough no foot bones. Fossilized knees and leg bones indicate that these hominids were fully adapted bipeds. *Homo sapiens,* our species, appeared sometime between 400,000 and 300,000 years ago. Early humans made their first appearance from 150,000 to 40,000 years before the present day, including the Neanderthal. Neanderthals were fully erect bipeds very similar to modern man. Although they differed from *Homo sapiens* considerably, their fossilized foot bones are indistinguishable from modern man's. Neanderthals died out about 40,000 years ago, when fully evolved modern man *(Homo sapiens sapiens)* was becoming widespread throughout the world.

In order to accomplish a fully erect posture and habitual bipedalism, the monkeylike foot of our ancestors was completely redesigned. The human foot differs from that of other primates. Our feet have both a longitudinal arch and a transverse arch. The transverse arch is in the area of the front of the foot at the metatarsal heads. Some living primates have a very slight longitudinal arch, but none has a transverse arch. The arches, along with the powerful ligamentous structures, allow for efficient weight distribution during gait. The modern foot is a rigid structure with very tight ligaments. Other primates have more flexible and muscular feet. The use of the foot as a grasping organ was completely abandoned in favor of efficient weight transmission.

The hand has always been considered a complicated structure, where in reality it is essentially a typical primate hand not terribly modified from earlier models. It is the foot that has evolved from a primitive handlike apparatus to the elegantly complex, superbly designed organ that it is today. Unfortunately it is often the most neglected part of the human body.

When thinking in evolutionary time frames, you can see what a recent event is the use of shoes. The poorly shod foot is subjected to all sorts of traumatic insults and has not had a chance to adapt to our modern ways.

My Waddyacallit Is Killing Me:
Terminology and Anatomy

The hipbone's connected to the knee bone's connected to the ankle bone's connected to the foot bone. If only it were that simple. It's not that the knee bone isn't connected to the anklebone or the anklebone to the foot bone. These are, indirectly, connected. If they were not, we'd all go to pieces. Unfortunately there's a lot of complicated stuff in between. In order to understand the many problems that affect the human foot, there are some basic terms, anatomical locations, and structures with which you must become familiar.

This is one of these nuts-and-bolts chapters mentioned in the introduction. It can be referred to while reading other chapters on specific foot problems. Simple line drawings are used to make what can be a very difficult subject easier to digest. There are some definitions of terms such as *medial, lateral, dorsal, plantar,* and so forth, but their locations are clearly identified on the drawings in this chapter and throughout the book. Drawings associated with specific problems appear in the text. Here we need discuss only

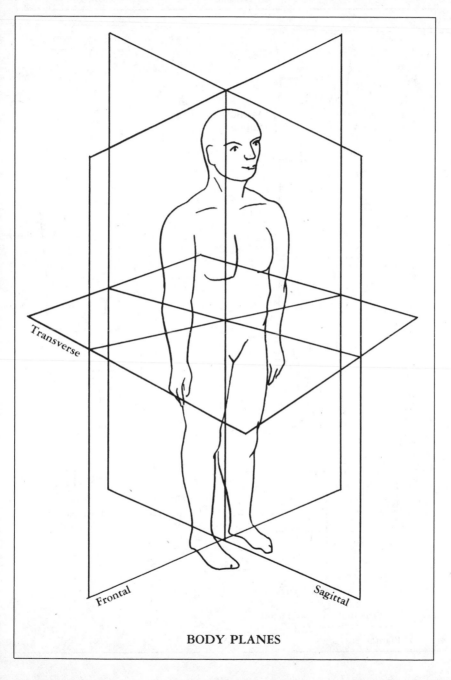

BODY PLANES

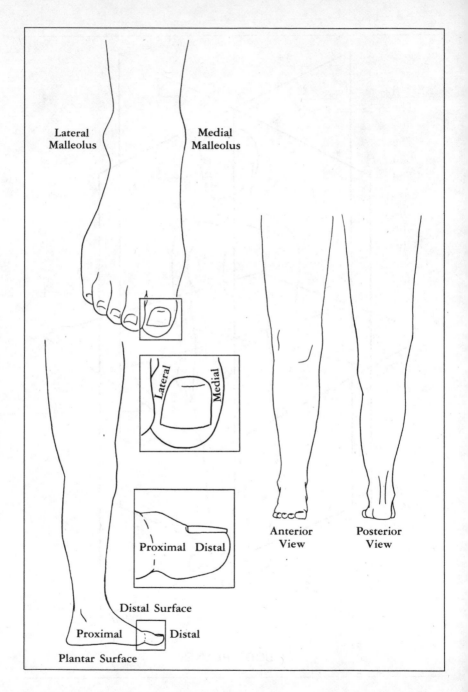

Lateral
Malleolus

Medial
Malleolus

Lateral

Medial

Proximal Distal

Distal Surface

Proximal   Distal

Plantar Surface

Anterior
View

Posterior
View

those terms required for the drawings to make sense. It is hoped that the drawings that follow will be worth thousands of words.

The *frontal plane* divides the body from top to bottom into a front section and a back section.

The *sagittal plane* divides the body from top to bottom into a left side and a right side.

The *transverse plane* divides the body going from side to side into a top part and a bottom part.

The *dorsal aspect* is on the top of the foot.

The *plantar aspect* is on the bottom of the foot.

The *medial aspect* is on the inside of the foot.

The *lateral aspect* is on the outside of the foot.

Both sets of terms tend to be confusing until you have encountered them a few times because it is always necessary to remember that they are *part-specific.* For example, what most patients think of as the inside of the big toe is in fact the lateral side because it is the part of the big toe closer to the outside of the foot.

Anterior describes a location in the front and forward. Your face.

Posterior describes a location toward the rear or behind. Your bum.

Proximal denotes a location closer to a point of reference. Your ankle is more proximal to your body than your big toe is.

Distal denotes a location farther from a point of reference. Your big toe is more distal to your body than your ankle is.

Superficial denotes a location near the surface. Your skin.

Deep denotes a location far beneath the surface. Bones.

There are six motions of the foot:

Dorsiflexion: Backward bending. The top of the foot bends toward the leg.

Plantar flexion: Forward-downward bending. The bottom of the foot bends toward the floor.

Adduction: Drawing the foot toward the median of the body. The foot goes toward the other foot.

Abduction: Drawing the foot away from the median of the body. The foot goes toward the outside.

Inversion: Raising the medial arch upward off the floor. (This includes supination and heightened longitudinal arch, adduction of the forefoot, and a degree of plantar flexion.)

Eversion: Raising the lateral side of the foot upward off the floor. (This includes pronation and lowered longitudinal arch, abduction of the forefoot, and a degree of dorsiflexion.)

A *pronated* foot will have a lowered longitudinal arch and a *supinated* foot will have a higher longitudinal arch.

The *bones* provide the skeletal structure of the foot. They are the framework on which all other tissues hang. There are twenty-eight bones in each foot (if you include the two sesamoid bones on the plantar aspect of the first metatarsal head), fourteen phalanges, five metatarsals, and seven tarsal bones.

Bone is by far the hardest element in the human body. Its exterior is harder than its interior cancellous part. Bone is covered by periosteum, a fibrous membrane that delivers the blood supply through periosteal vessels. There is no periosteum over the joint surfaces where the bones articulate. These areas are covered instead by articular cartilage, with a nonvascular structure. Muscles, tendons, and ligaments are attached to bone incorporated in the periosteum.

The classification of most bones is based on the bones' anatomical function and shape. The *long bones* possess the properties required for weight bearing and locomotion. Even small bones like the metatarsals are long bones because of their shape. *Short bones,* of which the tarsal bones are examples, facilitate balance and locomotion. *Flat bones,* such as the skull, pelvis, and sternum, serve protective functions.

The cavities of bones are filled with *marrow.* Marrow comes in two colors, yellow and red. The former, consisting mostly of fat cells, is found in the long bones. The latter, located in flat and short bones, is the source of blood cells. A cross section of a long

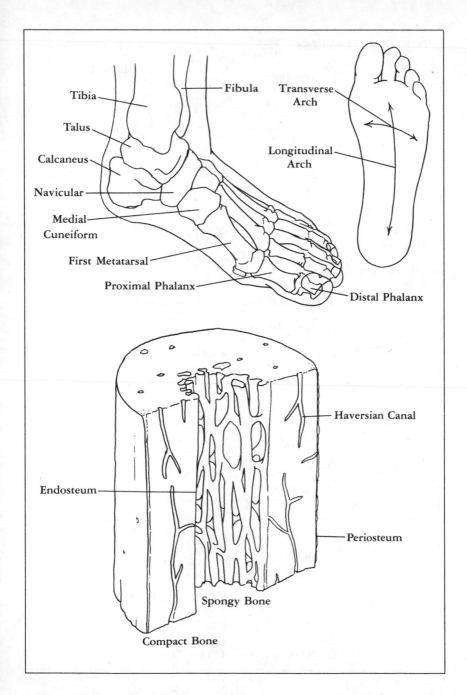

Tibia

Fibula

Transverse Arch

Talus

Calcaneus

Longitudinal Arch

Navicular

Medial Cuneiform

First Metatarsal

Proximal Phalanx

Distal Phalanx

Haversian Canal

Endosteum

Periosteum

Spongy Bone

Compact Bone

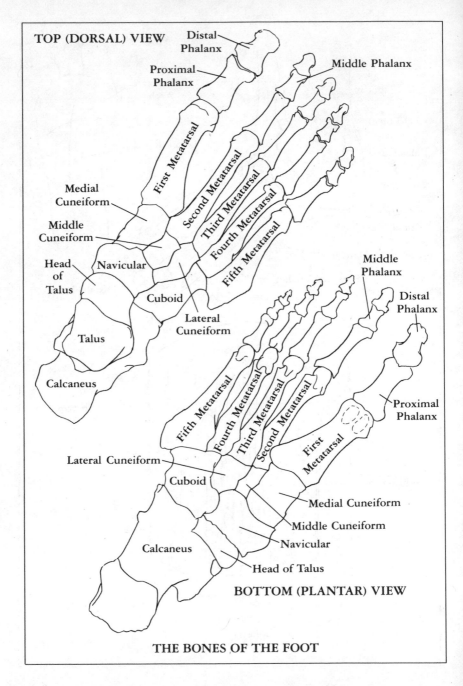

TOP (DORSAL) VIEW

Distal Phalanx

Proximal Phalanx

Middle Phalanx

First Metatarsal

Second Metatarsal

Third Metatarsal

Fourth Metatarsal

Fifth Metatarsal

Medial Cuneiform

Middle Cuneiform

Head of Talus

Navicular

Cuboid

Lateral Cuneiform

Talus

Calcaneus

Fifth Metatarsal

Fourth Metatarsal

Third Metatarsal

Second Metatarsal

First Metatarsal

Middle Phalanx

Distal Phalanx

Proximal Phalanx

Lateral Cuneiform

Cuboid

Medial Cuneiform

Middle Cuneiform

Navicular

Head of Talus

Calcaneus

BOTTOM (PLANTAR) VIEW

THE BONES OF THE FOOT

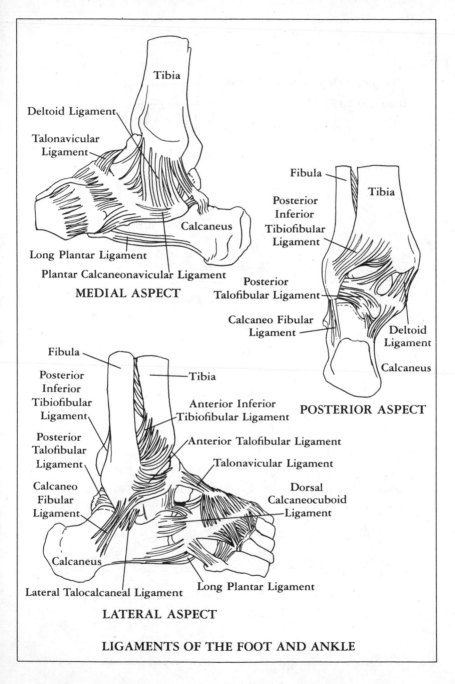

Tibia

Deltoid Ligament

Talonavicular
Ligament

Calcaneus

Long Plantar Ligament

Plantar Calcaneonavicular Ligament

MEDIAL ASPECT

Fibula

Tibia

Posterior
Inferior
Tibiofibular
Ligament

Posterior
Talofibular Ligament

Calcaneo Fibular
Ligament

Deltoid
Ligament

Calcaneus

POSTERIOR ASPECT

Fibula

Tibia

Posterior
Inferior
Tibiofibular
Ligament

Anterior Inferior
Tibiofibular Ligament

Posterior
Talofibular
Ligament

Anterior Talofibular Ligament

Talonavicular Ligament

Calcaneo
Fibular
Ligament

Dorsal
Calcaneocuboid
Ligament

Calcaneus

Lateral Talocalcaneal Ligament

Long Plantar Ligament

LATERAL ASPECT

LIGAMENTS OF THE FOOT AND ANKLE

35

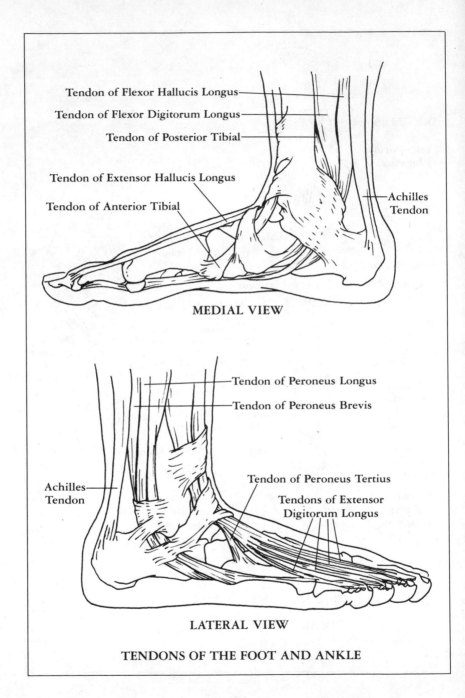

Tendon of Flexor Hallucis Longus

Tendon of Flexor Digitorum Longus

Tendon of Posterior Tibial

Tendon of Extensor Hallucis Longus

Tendon of Anterior Tibial

Achilles Tendon

MEDIAL VIEW

Tendon of Peroneus Longus

Tendon of Peroneus Brevis

Achilles Tendon

Tendon of Peroneus Tertius

Tendons of Extensor Digitorum Longus

LATERAL VIEW

TENDONS OF THE FOOT AND ANKLE

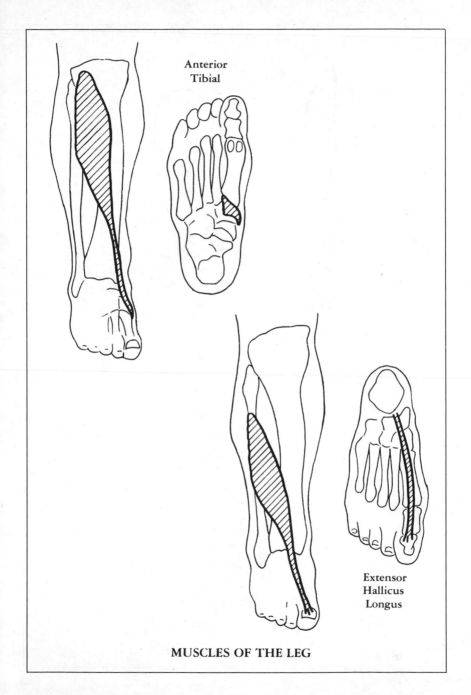

Anterior
Tibial

Extensor
Hallicus
Longus

MUSCLES OF THE LEG

37

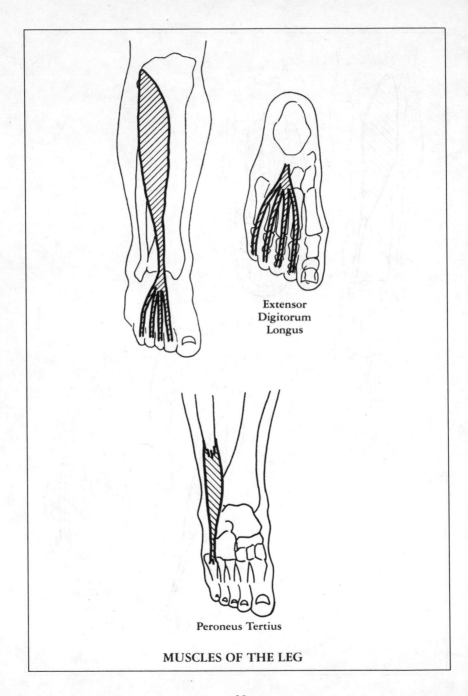

Extensor
Digitorum
Longus

Peroneus Tertius

MUSCLES OF THE LEG

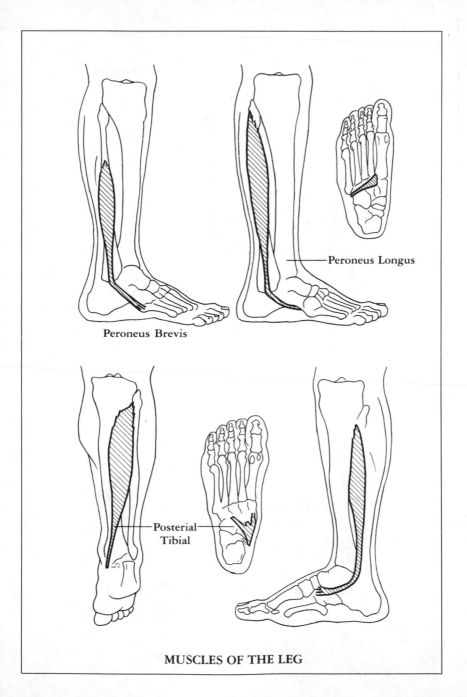

Peroneus Longus

Peroneus Brevis

Posterial
Tibial

MUSCLES OF THE LEG

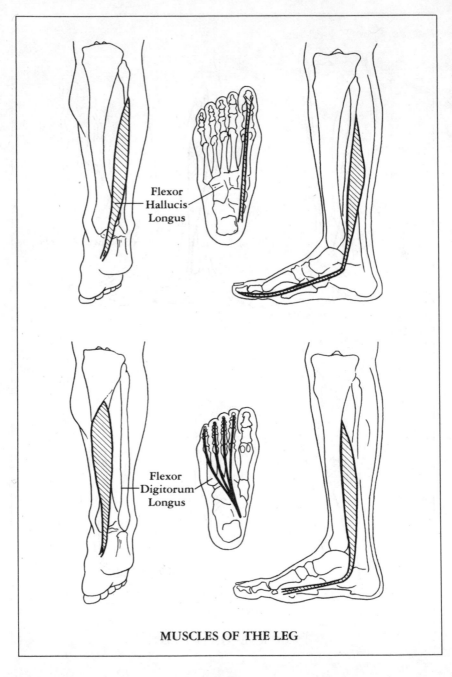

Flexor
Hallucis
Longus

Flexor
Digitorum
Longus

MUSCLES OF THE LEG

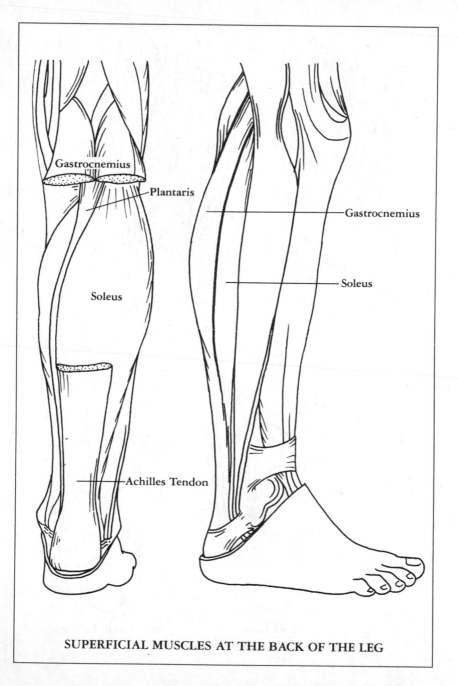

Gastrocnemius

Plantaris

Soleus

Achilles Tendon

Gastrocnemius

Soleus

SUPERFICIAL MUSCLES AT THE BACK OF THE LEG

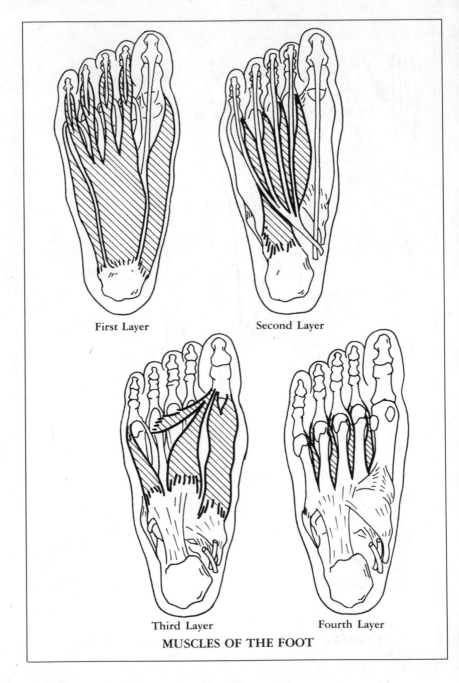

First Layer

Second Layer

Third Layer

Fourth Layer

MUSCLES OF THE FOOT

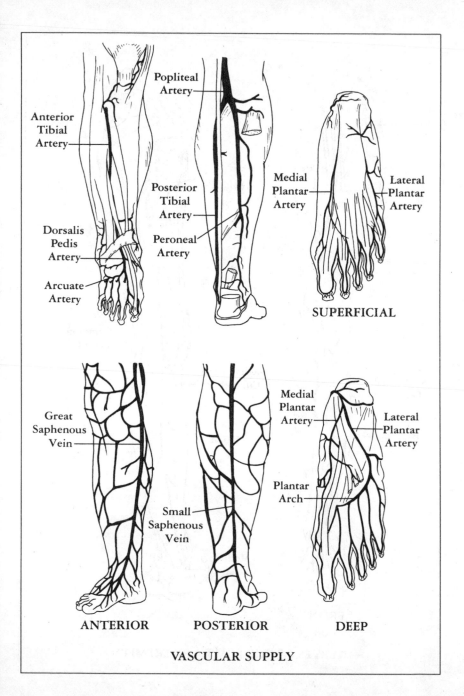

SUPERFICIAL

Anterior Tibial Artery

Dorsalis Pedis Artery

Arcuate Artery

Popliteal Artery

Posterior Tibial Artery

Peroneal Artery

Medial Plantar Artery

Lateral Plantar Artery

Great Saphenous Vein

Small Saphenous Vein

Medial Plantar Artery

Lateral Plantar Artery

Plantar Arch

ANTERIOR   POSTERIOR   DEEP

VASCULAR SUPPLY

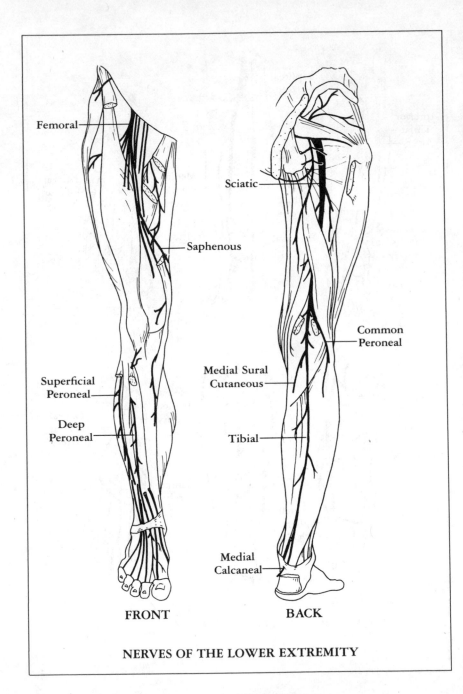

Femoral

Saphenous

Superficial
Peroneal

Deep
Peroneal

FRONT

Sciatic

Common
Peroneal

Medial Sural
Cutaneous

Tibial

Medial
Calcaneal

BACK

NERVES OF THE LOWER EXTREMITY

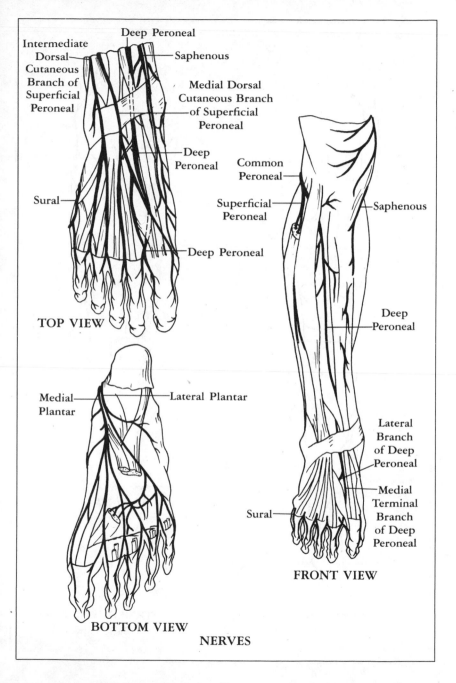

Intermediate Dorsal Cutaneous Branch of Superficial Peroneal

Deep Peroneal

Saphenous

Medial Dorsal Cutaneous Branch of Superficial Peroneal

Deep Peroneal

Sural

Deep Peroneal

TOP VIEW

Common Peroneal

Superficial Peroneal

Saphenous

Deep Peroneal

Medial Plantar

Lateral Plantar

Lateral Branch of Deep Peroneal

Medial Terminal Branch of Deep Peroneal

Sural

BOTTOM VIEW

FRONT VIEW

NERVES

45

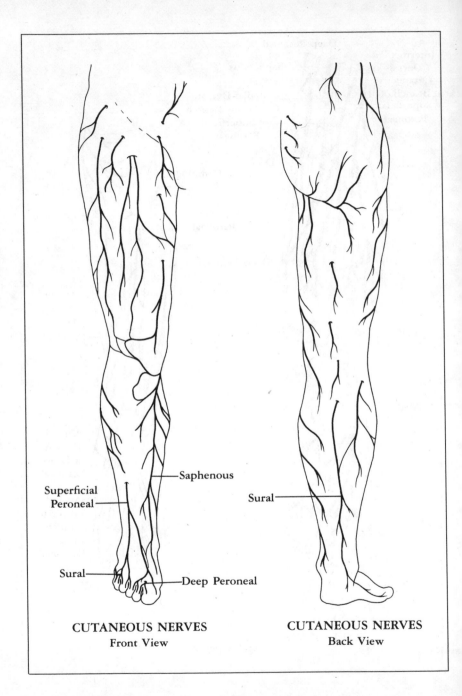

Saphenous

Superficial
Peroneal

Sural

Deep Peroneal

Sural

CUTANEOUS NERVES
Front View

CUTANEOUS NERVES
Back View

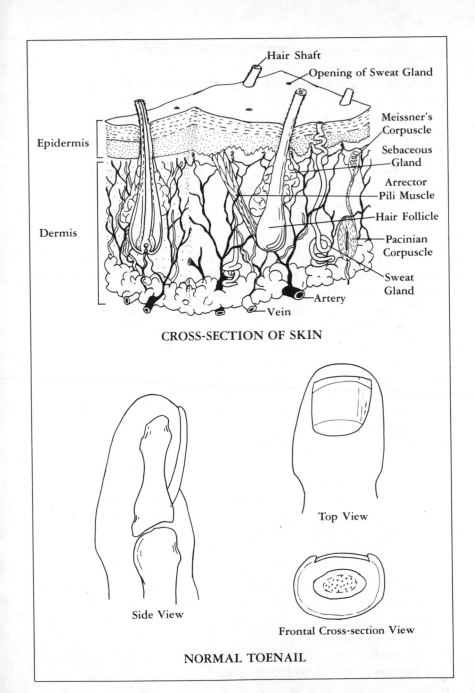

Hair Shaft

Opening of Sweat Gland

Meissner's Corpuscle

Sebaceous Gland

Arrector Pili Muscle

Hair Follicle

Pacinian Corpuscle

Sweat Gland

Epidermis

Dermis

Artery

Vein

CROSS-SECTION OF SKIN

Top View

Side View

Frontal Cross-section View

NORMAL TOENAIL

bone such as a metatarsal can demonstrate many of the interesting features of bone.

The joints and ligaments of the foot and ankle. The ligaments are thick, fibrous bands of tissue. They combine great strength with great flexibility. The fascial ligaments of the foot and ankle bind tendons of muscles coming from the leg to the foot. The four fascial ligaments are on the front and sides of the foot and ankle.

The *ankle* is a hinge joint composed of the lower end of the fibula (the lateral malleolus), the lower end of the tibia (the medial malleolus), and the upper portion of the talus. The joint is held together by the deltoid ligament, the anterior talo fibular, the posterior talo fibular, and the calcaneo fibular. This information will be important in the chapter on the injured foot.

The principal ligaments of the foot are the *long plantar,* the *short plantar,* and a fascial structure called the *plantar fascia.*

The *muscles* that act upon the foot come in two types: extrinsic and intrinsic. The former are the muscles that arise in the leg and insert into the foot. The latter are those that both arise and insert into the foot. The only muscle on the top of the foot is the extensor digitorum brevis. There are some dorsal interossei muscles, but they are between the metatarsals and considered with the fourth layer of muscles on the bottom of the foot.

The skin, technically known as the integument, covers the body, keeps deeper tissues from drying out, and protects vital organs from invasion by unwanted organisms and injury. The skin contains the sensory nerves that detect touch, temperature, position, and pain. It plays a crucial role in regulating body temperature and has an excretory and absorbing function.

The skin is composed of two layers, the epidermis, which is nonvascular and outermost, and the dermis beneath. Skin color is due to a pigment in the epidermis called melanin. The appendages of the skin are the nails, hair, sebaceous glands (of which there are very few in the feet), and the sweat glands.

Congratulations to any reader who has made it this far. Be assured that it is all downhill from here.

Do It Right!:
General Tips on Care of the Feet

1. Don't smoke. Surprise! You probably would not have guessed that this would top the list. This is probably the biggest favor that you can do for your feet (and your whole body). Smoking has a devastating effect on your circulation and on your body in general, so why not give yourself a big boost and stop smoking.

2. Keep walking. Walking is good exercise for the feet and improves the circulation. Psychologically it is important to maintain independence no matter what your age. So give your feet a workout every day and keep fit.

3. Inspect your feet visually every day. Look them over carefully for blisters, cracks between the toes, cuts, areas of redness, areas of abnormal shoe irritation, and nail problems. This is especially important for the person with circulatory problems and for diabetics. If you are too stiff to bend your feet for a proper inspection, use a mirror to examine the bottom of the feet.

4. Wash your feet daily in warm (not hot!) water using a mild

soap. Do not rub with a rough towel. Dry carefully between the toes. If you draw a towel too aggressively between the toes, you can crack the skin and end up with an infection. Follow the careful cleansing and drying of your feet with the application of a cream or lotion of a lanolin base. This will help maintain moisture and help with dry skin. Do not use between the toes. If you have a perspiration problem, you can dust the feet with any of the commercially available foot powders.

5. Avoid temperature extremes. When you have a neuropathy or poor circulation, the skin of the foot is considerably less sensitive, and extremes of temperature may not be noticed. If you have a lessened sensitivity to hot and cold, you should test bath water with an elbow or have a family member do it for you. Besides scalding from bath water, one must be careful with hot-water bottles and heating pads. It is a good rule not to use these devices on the feet. Do not use below the knee. If your feet are cold at night, it is safer to use woolen socks to keep them warm. Never place your feet on a heat register. Do not walk barefoot, as there are many hazards awaiting the unshod foot. Never walk on hot surfaces, such as those beautiful white, tempting sandy beaches, or around swimming pools.

6. Do not use strong chemical agents for the removal of corns and callouses. This includes medicated corn pads. Never attempt to cut corns and callouses yourself. One wrong move and you can cut the skin and end up with a serious infection. Diabetics and patients with impaired circulation have to be especially careful and must seek professional care for their foot problems.

7. Nails should be cut straight across. Do not cut the nail shorter than the fleshy part of the toe and do not curve the sides of the nails. Do not dig into the corners or along the nail groove. You should not cut your nails with scissors and never use a knife or razor blades. If the nails tend to grow in, a very small piece of cotton inserted in the corners can sometimes help. If tissue around the nail is injured, the application of an alcohol swab can cleanse

the area. Cleansing with a soft brush will remove accumulations of dead tissue in the nail groove. Discolorations, abnormal nail growth, and unusual thickness should be called to the attention of your podiatrist.

8. Inspect the inside of shoes daily for exposed nails, cracks, torn lining, and foreign objects. Even foot powders can accumulate and cake and cause an irritation. Shoes should not be worn without stockings. Thongs and sandals are not good for your feet. It is a good idea to change your shoes during the day; that way you are never in any one pair long enough to cause serious damage. Take an extra pair along to work. Remember, the proper shoe for the proper occasion. Shoes should feel comfortable at the time of purchase. If they do not, they will probably not feel any better later on. Buy shoes in the afternoon after the feet have had a chance to swell a little. Wear new shoes a couple of hours at a time for the first four or five days to give them a chance to break in properly. Never buy shoes with corrective pads or buildups without the advice of your podiatrist.

9. Wear properly fitted stockings without thick seams. Be sure to leave room at the tip of the foot while standing for a proper fit. If you get a hole in your sock, throw it out. Mended areas can cause irritations to sensitive skin. Change stockings daily. Stockings should be washed and then rinsed carefully to remove excess soap. Natural fibers such as cotton and wool absorb moisture better than artificial fibers. Never wear garters. They constrict blood vessels and impair circulation.

10. It is important for travelers to pack shoes that fit. This is not a time to try out a new pair of shoes. Keep in mind the climate of your destination. In warmer areas the feet tend to swell more, and in areas with colder weather heavier stockings may be in order. If you are traveling by plane, take your shoes off as soon as you sit down and change into a comfortable travel slipper. Exercise can help relieve stiffness associated with long journeys. Extend your legs and point your toes for a few minutes. Lift your feet and rotate in circles in each direction fifteen or twenty times.

11. If your feet hurt or you are concerned about any abnormality, see your podiatrist. Many cities and towns have a referral service run by the local podiatry society. It is possible a friend or relative may use a podiatrist to whom they could refer you. Most family practitioners and internists will refer their more complicated foot problems to a podiatrist, and they can provide you with a list of names. When you find a podiatrist, make sure you feel absolutely comfortable with your choice. If you do not, get another one. There are plenty of very good doctors around and a few bad ones. Make sure you get one of the former. Your podiatrist should be a member of the American Podiatric Medical Association.

Buy Right!:
Information and Tips
Regarding Shoes

Man has worn shoes for millennia. Egyptians wore sandals fashioned out of papyrus leaves. The Japanese, the Greeks, and the ancient Romans all wore sandals of one type or another, some of them quite beautiful. In the colder regions the Eskimos and Indians made foot coverings from animal skins for both warmth and protection. In Renaissance times throughout Europe shoes were common among the upper classes, the fashions often ridiculous. A differentiated right and left shoe first made its appearance in the middle of the nineteenth century. Until that time shoes were made from a straight last.

A shoe last is basically a reproduction of the human foot over which shoes are made. Lasts increase one-third inch in length and one-quarter inch in width between sizes. It is very important to remember that shoe sizes vary slightly from manufacturer to manufacturer; therefore you may not always take the same numerical size and width all the time. A size 10D of one make may feel just fine while a 10D from another make may not. It is also important to use a little common sense when selecting shoes.

Shoes should be tried on for fit in the afternoon, as the feet swell during the day.

Remember to wear the proper shoe style for the proper occasion. If you are getting dressed up for an important function, by all means wear a stylish shoe. If, however, you plan to go shopping and will be on your feet for an extended period of time, wear something a little less stylish with more support.

The principal parts of the shoe are the upper, the insole, the outsole, and the heel. The ball of the shoe refers to the area of the metatarsal heads. The shank is the area between the heel and the ball of the shoe. The shank helps reinforce the arch and is usually made of steel, steel and leather, or wood. The forepart of the shoe is the part extending from the ball to the ends of the toes. The extreme forepart of the shoe is called the tip, and the vertical height of the shoe in the area of the toes is called the toe box. The area behind the tip is called the vamp, which extends backward over the ball and instep and then joins to the back and sides of the upper.

Women's shoes have been responsible for many forefoot problems such as hammer toes and bunions. Shoe fit is extremely important, as one must have adequate length and width for the weight-bearing foot. Hand-me-down shoes are a very bad idea. A shoe must conform to the shape of the individual's foot and should be shaped to the width of the heel and the width of the forefoot. Flexibility of the sole of the shoe allows the metatarsophalangeal joints to function properly. Heels should be of moderate height, approximately one and one-half inches, and are ideally made of rubber. Leather is the best upper material, as it breathes, preventing burning and unusual perspiration. Plastic does not work well at all, and plastic shoes should be avoided.

Because the foot is one of the most vulnerable parts of the body, it is subject to a variety of industrial hazards. Safety shoes have been a valuable contribution to industrial health. Shoes with steel

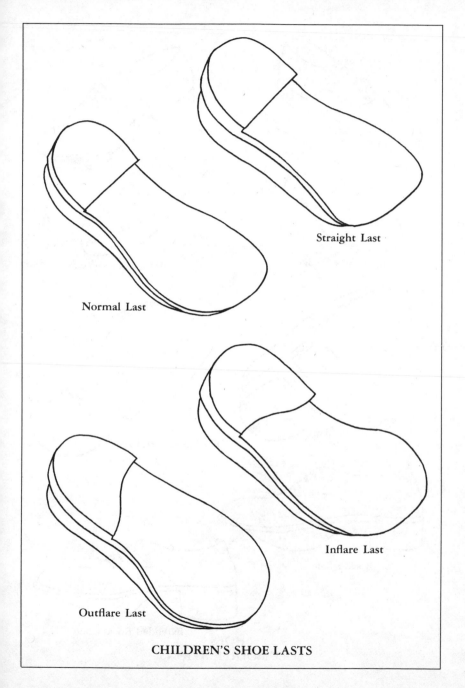

Straight Last

Normal Last

Inflare Last

Outflare Last

CHILDREN'S SHOE LASTS

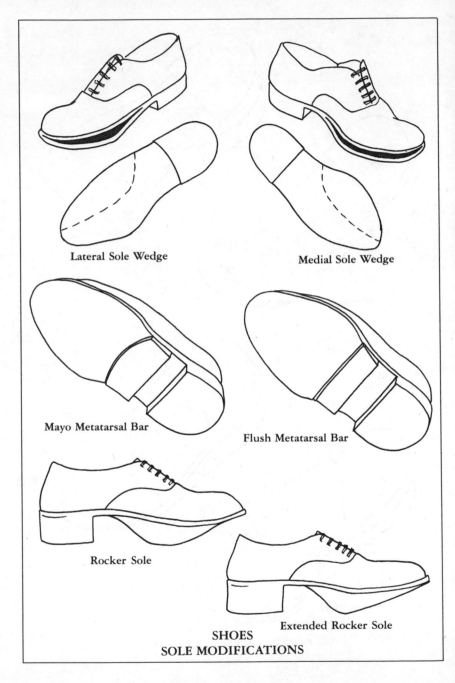

Lateral Sole Wedge

Medial Sole Wedge

Mayo Metatarsal Bar

Flush Metatarsal Bar

Rocker Sole

Extended Rocker Sole

SHOES
SOLE MODIFICATIONS

toe caps are available, as are shoes designed to dissipate static electricity to the ground, thereby preventing ignition of explosive materials. Electrical-hazard shoes are intended to provide protection against open circuits of less than 600 volts under dry conditions. Shoes are available with puncture-resistant and chemically resistant soles.

The manufacture of children's shoes is very big business. Most doctors feel that an infant whose feet are in a neutral position does not need shoes and requires bootees only for warmth. Footgear is really not essential until a child begins to walk. In the prewalking stage a very soft leather shoe may be worn. In the early walking phase a semisoft, flexible-outsole-type shoe is best. The upper should be soft and flexible. At first a high-top style shoe is recommended to aid in stabilizing the ankle. At between twenty to thirty months of age the child can be transferred to a low shoe. There are different types of corrective shoes available for children. Aside from the conventional-last shoes, which are standard from heel to toe and have a right and left, there are straight lasts, outflare lasts, and inflare lasts. A straight-last shoe is just that: It is straight from heel to toe and the shoes are interchangeable. Outflare lasts are used when the forefoot is going inward in a condition called metatarsus adductus. The outflare forces the foot outward. Inflare lasts force the foot inward and are used to maintain correction after treatment for pronated feet.

There are many modifications that can be made to both the inside and the outside of the shoe. Wedges and pads are used to accomplish some of them. A wedge is usually made of leather and placed on the exterior walking surface or within the shoe's construction. A wedge is intended to alter the weight-bearing pattern of the foot. Pads are used inside the shoe and are usually made of felt. They work on specific spots of the foot.

Modifications can be made in the heel area, as in the case of Thomas heels, heel lifts, widened heels, and SACH heels. A Thomas heel is the most commonly used. It brings the heel bone, the calcaneus, from a valgus position to a more neutral one. It is

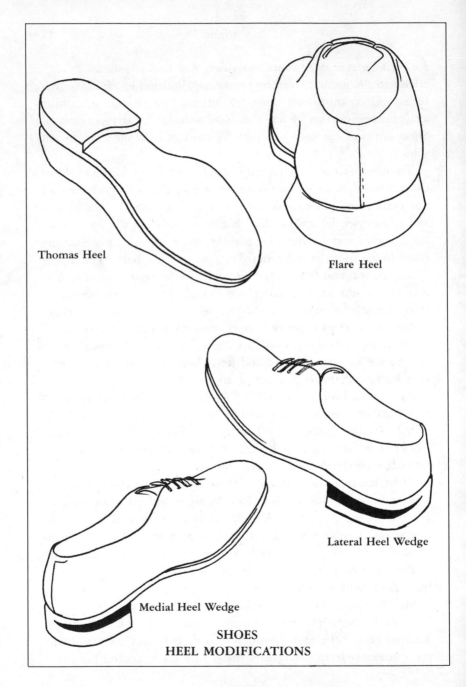

Thomas Heel

Flare Heel

Lateral Heel Wedge

Medial Heel Wedge

**SHOES
HEEL MODIFICATIONS**

never used if the heel bone is in a varus position. It consists of a flaring or forward extension of the inside of the heel.

A heel lift also can be used to tilt the heel bone, depending upon on which side of the heel the lift is placed. It is usually between three and six centimeters in thickness, with a feathered edge.

Widened heels are used to help stabilize the subtalar joint in the rear part of the foot.

A SACH heel is an elevated soft heel that will cushion the impact of initial ground contact.

A variety of wedges and bars used to treat many different types of conditions can be added to the sole of the shoe. A wedge or lift in the region of the great toe can make the toe less flexible and restrict motion. (The condition of hallux rigidus is treated this way.) A metatarsal bar can be placed on the outside of the sole just behind the metatarsal heads in order to transfer weight away from this area. Metatarsal bars are used to treat problems such as a diminished fat pad in the bottom of the foot, Morton's syndrome, and painful callouses. The Denver bar and the Hauser bar are used to treat metatarsalgia. A Rocker sole is used to limit weight bearing on the forefoot.

Many different types of foot pads can be placed in the shoe to help alleviate the symptoms of a myriad of foot problems. Felt or foam-rubber heel lifts can cushion heel spurs on the bottom of the heel. A painful posterior heel problem can be helped by heel pads to elevate the foot out of the shoe, eliminating pressure. Metatarsal pads, if properly placed, can help metatarsalgia and neuromas. Pads with apertures cut in them can protect calloused areas of the foot.

With the increased interest in health and fitness there has been a corresponding increase in sports-related injuries related to footgear. There are many different shoes available for specific sports, and they are generally very good, but there are a number of things to look for when selecting a shoe for your sport. In general we get what we pay for, so avoid the cheap imports whenever possible.

When selecting a shoe for basketball, a hightop is the first choice. A hightop shoe can be very helpful in preventing ankle injuries, the most common injury associated with the sport.

Tennis is frequently played by the weekend athlete. A tennis shoe must provide traction on a variety of surfaces from asphalt to clay. The shoe must be durable to resist abrasion caused by toe drag, and be well cushioned.

Running shoes should have both outsole and insole cushions, along with lightweight, comfortable uppers that breathe and extended heel counters made of a firm material. The shoe must also be flexible. See the chapter on running for more information. There is also a section on walking shoes in the walking chapter.

Cleated footwear worn for soccer, football, and baseball must have adequate cushioning. Cleats should not be more than three inches apart.

Aerobic shoes need adequate cushioning and should give good support.

The most important thing to remember is that each sport demands a specific shoe, and one should carefully research any purchase to be sure the shoe you select provides the proper environment for the foot during participation in your given sport.

With the advent of orthotics, shoe therapy has become a less popular method of treatment. Orthotics are devices, made of a variety of materials, that are used to place the foot in proper balance. They are obtained by first taking an impression of the feet in a corrected position. This impression is filled with a substance, usually plaster, and a model of the foot is created. This model is often corrected further. An orthotic is fabricated over this corrected model. The orthotic is portable and can be transferred from shoe to shoe. It looks something like an old-fashioned arch support. It is usually rigid, but can be flexible also. It should be obtained from a podiatrist trained in the biomechanics of the foot. It may look very simple but is a very sophisticated device.

Molded shoes have been around for a long time and are very useful in treating patients with significant foot deformities, such as

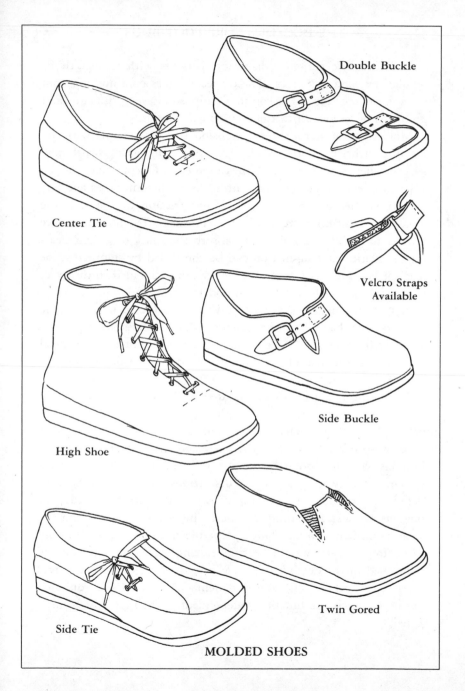

Double Buckle

Center Tie

Velcro Straps
Available

High Shoe

Side Buckle

Side Tie

Twin Gored

MOLDED SHOES

severely arthritic patients, diabetics, patients with leg-length irregularities, and amputees. These special shoes cure nothing, but
go a long way toward accommodating some very difficult foot
problems of various distortions and inadequacies.

Molded shoes offer a three-dimensional fit for patients with deforming arthritic problems. Besides providing exact width and
length, they give the added measurement of depth and can be
adapted to relieve pressure on painful flexed hammer toes and any
bony prominence. They reduce plantar friction by cradling the
foot, which in turn prevents plantar callosities. The plantar surface
can be made soft and yielding to absorb the shock of weight bearing. Pronation and supination can be controlled by stabilizing the
rearfoot heel area. A soft leather upper can be molded to the exact
dimension of the foot to accommodate corns and bunion deformities. They can be made with a Velcro closure to help arthritic
patients with badly deformed hands. Molded shoes are especially
good for the insensitive foot of the diabetic. The three-dimensional
fit ensures fewer areas of friction that could produce dangerous diabetic foot ulcers.

Limb length can be accommodated easily with the discrepancy
built directly into the shoe. People with severe pes cavus or pes
valgo planus (high arch and no arch) type feet benefit from this
type of shoe also. People with extremely painful and deformed
bunions who are absolutely not surgical candidates due to serious
systemic disease can have these distortions adequately accommodated with a molded shoe. Amputees do well with them, too, for
obvious reasons. The stump can be cushioned and padded and the
shoe molded in a cosmetically acceptable manner. These shoes are
made from a semi-weight-bearing casting technique that can be
performed in the doctor's office. While these shoes are expensive,
when one considers the added benefits of an otherwise disabled
person being able to function independently, the high cost is miti-
gated.

Left Right, Left Right:
The Essentials of Walking

After reading about the multitude of afflictions that take aim at your feet, you might come to the conclusion that God put those flippers at the ends of our legs simply to give us grief.

The feet are, as you may have noticed, an absolute requirement for the oldest and most basic form of human locomotion, walking. For most of human history, walking was seen as a necessary means to get to a destination. It never occurred to anyone to think of it as a virtue in its own right. But this has changed. Concomitant with the advent of jogging as a sport, walking has come to be seen as a source of pleasure and a tolerable form of exercise. There are presently over four million Americans who see themselves as serious walkers and who have demonstrably benefited from their new pastime.

Many of these people discovered the convenience and inexpensiveness of walking only after spending thousands of dollars on high-tech equipment whose learning curve was longer than its ability to maintain interest. Walking is a low-impact sport, which reduces the chance of bone, joint, and muscle injuries. It provides all the benefits of other aerobic high-impact sports, and is probably the safest way to burn fat and keep it off. An excellent way to get fit and stay fit. If you have a serious debility that precludes hoisting heavy weights, dancing to death in front of your TV, or in some similar way assaulting your body, walking permits the advantages of exercise without the threat of harm. Many diabetics and heart patients, for example, have seen their health and happiness blossom when they took to walking under a doctor's supervision.

Others have discovered that walking is a wonderful adjunct to a diet. It burns fat while it tightens muscle. While walking might not turn you into an Arnold Schwarzenegger, it can keep you fit, firm, and happy. Walking permits you to burn as many calories as jogging (though it takes a bit longer), and those calories are not lost at the expense of your joints. A hundred calories per mile of walking may not seem like much. However, a three-mile walk each day will, other things being equal, amount to a loss of thirty-five pounds a year. At the very least this means that you easily balance the tendency to gain weight with age.

And there are other bonuses. Walking is an antidote to stress. It makes you feel good and improves your performance at work and play. Walking has cured people of sleep problems of many years' duration.

As with any exercise, if you are over thirty-five you should get a medical evaluation before beginning a walking program. The odds are overwhelming that the doctor will encourage you to begin. But there are individuals for whom walking is not indicated, and you want to be certain you are not one of them.

The names given to various types of walking are many, depending on time, region, and the like. But all of these basically fall under one of three classes of walking: race walking, fitness walking, and regular walking.

You know race walking. It's that sport that gives new meaning to the word *silly*. Rules requiring a gait that makes the race walker look like a ruptured chicken. One foot must at all times be in contact with the ground, with the leg straight as the body passes over it. This forces an exaggerated hip motion and a pumping action of arms that are held close to the body. Judges are rigid in their enforcement of the rules (as indeed they must be; no one would do anything that looks this silly if not forced to).

They may look a little ridiculous, but on the other hand, when was the last time you saw a fat race walker?

Race walking has been around for over a hundred years and has been an Olympic sport since 1908. About a quarter of the 45,000 members of the Walkers' Club of America are competitive race walkers.

Fitness walking is a catchall term for aerobic walking, health walking, power walking, and weight walking. Most serious walkers agree that the best technique consists of a gait in which one foot is placed directly in front of the other. This maximizes balance and smoothness.

Speed should not be overemphasized in fitness walking. Even moderate exercise of this type is associated with decreased rates of myocardial infarction and sudden death and with increased longevity. Studies consistently show that inactive adults are nearly twice as likely to develop coronary heart disease as are active adults—the same difference as between nonsmokers and pack-a-day smokers.

Fitness walking is not just for the elderly. While it was once thought that walking was insufficiently demanding to assist the young in keeping healthy, it is now clear that thirty minutes a day of 5.3-mph walking will enable a young person to attain the exercise target heart rate.

Our walking rate as we go about our daily activities is about three miles per hour. The average person needs to increase this by only about a third—to four miles per hour—in order to reach his desirable exercise heart rate. When he does this, he is no longer just walking but is engaging in a program of fitness walking. Not so hard, right?

The cardiovascular effects of such a program are immense. Because the legs are called upon to perform increased work, cardiac output and stroke volume are increased. Almost immediately upon beginning a fitness walk, you will find that your heart rate and respiration accelerate.

After a few minutes these level off and a steady state is achieved, and energy production becomes an issue of aerobic metabolism.

The short-term effects are a decrease in the resting heart rate and an increase in maximal oxygen consumption. In other words a given task can be accomplished using less oxygen and the heart doesn't have to work as hard.

We have referred to the long-term effects: The probability of heart disease decreases, weight drops, temperament improves, and attention can be given to other problems (like smoking). Indeed some people so enjoy the feeling of health they get from walking that they find they can give up other bad habits surprisingly easily. The average person burns only 20 to 25 percent fewer calories walking a mile than running one.

In the typical exercise program, over 60 percent of people drop out fairly early on. Very few drop out of fitness walking programs. This alone is a powerful argument for walking, since an exercise program you stop following is worthless, no matter what its inherent virtues. Fitness walking is the mainstay of virtually all cardiac rehabilitation programs.

So, you're convinced, right? Well, the first thing to do is have your doctor do an in-depth check to make sure you haven't developed any of the early signs of heart disease. A resting electrocardiogram is recommended. If you are over forty-five, or younger with a risk of coronary disease (a smoker, for example), a stress test is also advisable.

If you pass these tests (as nearly all of you will), you are capable of the initial demands of fitness walking: participation three to five days a week (fifteen to sixty minutes per session) and an intensity requiring your heart to work at greater than 70 percent of its maximum capability. A tremendous bonus associated with fitness walking is a marked decrease in the lipoprotein cholesterol level in the bloodstream. You can lower your risk of heart disease.

A smooth, steady pace is important to obtain your desired target heart rate for the most efficient cardiovascular aerobic workout. To ascertain your target heart rate, use the following formula. Doing so does not require a degree in number theory, but it is important to double-check your figures.

Subtract your age from 220. This is your maximum heart rate. Take your pulse for 60 seconds upon awakening. Subtract your pulse rate from your maximum heart rate. Multiply this number by 0.6. The result is your target *zone*. Add your pulse rate to your target zone. You now have your target heart rate. Divide by six for your 10-second target heart rate. Take your pulse while walking, for 10 seconds. If your pulse is less than your 10-second target heart rate, increase your pace. If your pulse is faster than your 10-second heart rate, decrease your pace.

Before you begin to walk, it is a good idea to perform stretching movements for about five minutes. For example you can stretch your calf (and preclude the possibility of a cramp) by doing a simple calf stretch: Place the back foot to the ground and bend the foot. Both knees should be forward. Hold this position for about thirty seconds.

The quadriceps stretch entails pulling your foot toward your buttocks with the opposite hand while keeping the knee pointing straight to the ground. For a hamstring stretch, place a heel on an elevated surface (such as a stair) with the upper knee slightly bent and the back straight. Carefully lean forward from the hips with the hands extended toward the ankle.

Always remember to be gentle. NEVER bounce or force yourself beyond your limits.

After you stretch, begin to walk—slowly. Do so for about five minutes in order to increase your heart rate. Now walk briskly for twenty-five minutes, keeping your target heart rate in mind. After about ten minutes check your pulse and adjust your pace up or down to make it equal your target rate.

As you gain experience, you will develop the style you are most

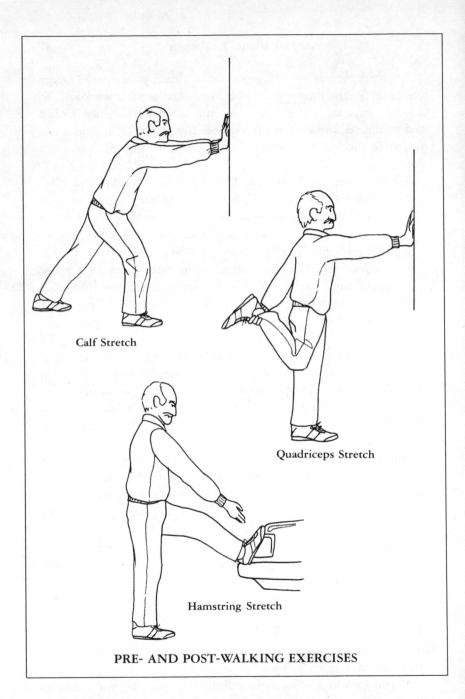

Calf Stretch

Quadriceps Stretch

Hamstring Stretch

PRE- AND POST-WALKING EXERCISES

comfortable with. However, whatever that style is, it should incorporate certain elements: You should move your arms and legs vigorously with your knees pointing forward; your hips should be even, your shoulders relaxed, and you should take deep, even breaths.

Your walk should end with a five-minute decrease in speed to facilitate cooling down and a five-minute stretching period to prevent stiffness and to increase flexibility.

Much has been made of the importance of the walking shoe. Half of this makes sense. The truth is, the difference between an adequate shoe and a great shoe is insignificant in every respect but cost. But the difference between a poor shoe and an adequate shoe is the difference between pain and pleasure.

It is always advisable to stick with a well-known brand. There *are* good off-brand shoes to be found, but it is difficult to tell when this is the case. Famous makers know that a truly poor shoe is disastrous for their reputation, so they can be counted on to meet at least a minimal standard.

The major companies each have twenty or more models, and the differences are real. The needs of a hundred-meter-dash man are different from those of a backcountry hiker. As a walker you will be looking for a shoe that combines ruggedness, comfort, and cushioning.

Most walkers whose careers do not prohibit doing so soon come to wear their walking shoes most of the day. They are simply far more comfortable than any more formal footwear. However, you can avail yourself of this comfort only by considering your choice of shoe carefully.

The first task is the easiest: Do not bother with special-purpose shoes not made for walking. Do not, for example, buy a shoe pitched as a racer. One-half ounce may be important to a world-class sprinter, but the loss of cushioning represented by the half ounce is much more important to you than the slight extra weight.

It may seem like a lot to have to weigh the advantages and disadvantages of laces, heel supports, soles, and arch supports. But you spend most of your life on your feet and in your shoes. They deserve the thought you would routinely give the purchase of a new television set. Most people spend about six hours a day on their feet and walk almost ten thousand steps!

Always shop for walking shoes (or, for that matter, any other shoes) in the afternoon. Your foot swells as you walk through the day, and the shoe bought in the morning will squeeze in the afternoon. Take socks of the type you will wear with the shoes and an old pair of shoes for comparison with the new.

Many things must be considered if a proper fit is to be attained, and even as minor a choice as that between lace and Velcro closures can be crucial. (Laces permit the shoe to conform to your feet point-by-point; Velcro acts as a vise when your foot expands.)

The more rugged the terrain you plan to walk, the more rugged the shoe you must buy. On the other hand there's no point in buying a shoe with heavy protection against snakes if you plan to amble down Main Street.

Once you have chosen to examine a pair of shoes, look inside. Check for any irregularities that could irritate your foot. If you can feel the irregularity with your hand, you can be certain it will abrade your foot.

To determine the proper length of a walking shoe, pinch the front of the shoe at the big toe with the width of your thumb. If the empty space is greater than the width of your thumb, the shoe is too long.

To determine the proper width, look closely at the lace holes. If they are more than, or less than, a thumb's width apart when the shoes are snugly laced, they are not for you.

If the shoe passes these tests, consider your intuitive response to it. If the shoe seems a little uncomfortable now, it *won't* get better. It's understandable that the inconvenience of trying on shoes (no one's idea of fun) makes you want to overlook slight problems, but trust us, the problems will seem anything but slight by the third mile.

Is there enough room in the front of the toes, both in the toe box and around the toes? Is there enough height in the instep above the arch? Is the arch of the shoe precisely where it should be, directly under your arch? Is the heel snug enough to guarantee stability without cramping? Stability without comfort becomes instability as you alter your step in a vain attempt to increase comfort.

Do not confuse a walking shoe with a running shoe. The two serve different purposes. When you walk, one foot is always in contact with the ground. As a result, when the heel strikes the ground, the pressure is gradually transferred to the rest of the foot. In running, both feet are off the ground simultaneously; the foot makes contact with three times the force, and the force is transmitted far more quickly. We will discuss this at greater length when we take a detailed look at gait.

Because the walker does not have to endure the forces involved in running, his shoe does not need the thick midsole characteristic of the running shoe. The thinner midsole permits a flexibility that allows the walking foot its natural heel-to-toe motion. The heel of a walking shoe, incidentally, should be lower in relationship to the forefoot than would be the case in a running shoe.

Good walking shoes come in a variety of materials. As long as the material is porous and sufficiently strong to give proper support, the choice comes down to the abrasion resistance and longevity of leather versus the lightness and greater porosity of synthetics, such as nylon.

It is always worthwhile to try shoes made by a few different manufacturers. Shoes of the "same" size vary considerably from brand to brand because no two manufacturers' lasts are identical.

Once you have determined that a shoe has all the criteria we have discussed, look for extra features. Highly desirable is a slit in the tongue through which you pass the laces. Removable insoles make possible the use of orthotics should these prove necessary. An absorbent lining will tend to keep your feet dry, a feature that is of particular interest to those with a tendency to blister or develop athlete's foot.

When you have worn a pair of shoes for a while and found them satisfactory, buy another, identical pair. Shoes last much longer when alternated, and the chances of contracting a fungus is decreased by the extra drying time.

Incidentally should your shoes get wet, do not force-dry them. Putting shoes next to the radiator to dry them superfast may seem like a nifty idea, but it is a death sentence for the little darlings. If the shoes are made of a synthetic material, simply let them dry naturally. If they are leather, do the same and follow the drying with saddle soap and a good moisturizing polish.

Important points to remember: a *proper fit*, a *lace-up shoe*, good *heel support*, a *flexible sole*, and a good *arch support*. Always try a shoe on before you buy it. Unusual wear patterns or abnormal shoe breakdown after purchase needs to be called to the attention of a professional.

You would think that, once your shoes have passed muster and you've done your stretching exercises and you're walking in good form, that's all there would be to worry about. Well, not quite. Walking is a simple exercise in that there is not much you have to do for success (other than walk of course), but it is less simple in the things you must avoid if you are to keep out of trouble.

For example, *never* wear ankle weights. It may seem sensible to increase the load, and thereby the efficiency of the exercise, by adding a couple of pounds to your ankles, but it's not. Two pounds of metal at the ankle makes about as much anatomical sense as a bowling ball at the elbow. They will put pressures on your joints that evolution never anticipated and are guaranteed to cause you problems.

Safe walking, like safe sex, is primarily a question of common sense. You wouldn't drive long distances without adding water to your car's radiator to keep your car cool, so don't take to the paths without a fully functioning cooling system. Drink from eight to ten glasses of water a day. Tap water is fine; fancy French stuff with bubbles doesn't do a thing for you that tap water doesn't.

If you walk at dawn, dusk, or night, wear light reflectors. The greatest threat to the health of a walker is the inattentive driver, and it behooves us to make him attentive. Reflectors won't do much against a nasty dog, but mailmen swear by those sprays that make you as attractive to a nasty dog as a nasty dog is to you.

There is a small but finite chance that a car or a dog or one of the other enemies of the walker will cause you harm or put you in danger. Thus you should always carry identification and a few quarters lest you have to phone for help.

Above all, do not walk if you have a sprain, blister, or other problem that will be made worse by walking, and stop walking *immediately* if you feel dizzy or develop pains in your chest or arms.

Power walking is an attempt to increase the benefits of walking by adding to the load. We have already mentioned that there are ways *not* to do this (putting weights on the ankles). Likewise, we are not fond of the current fashion for hand weights because it is too easy for the arm to swing in an unnatural motion. Weights on the hips or chest, on the other hand, are, if increased very gradually, an effective way of increasing the benefits of walking without adding to the time you must devote. Elderly patients and patients with cardiac problems, however, should never use weights, because the threat of raised blood pressure is too great. And, again, no one should *ever* use ankle weights.

Regular walking can be as satisfying and as much fun as any of the more demanding forms of walking. You can do it almost anytime and anywhere, and unlike baseball, you don't have to round up seventeen of your closest friends. The costs are limited and you don't have to spend hours studying the latest equipment; once you've got your shoes, you're ready to go. You needn't devote hours to practicing fancy techniques or wade through boring how-to books.

You can be a walker twenty seconds from now. (But make sure that you walk to a store that sells good athletic shoes and follow the directions given above.) If you are a couch potato whose idea of sport is turning on the tube, you can leave all that behind you with only a simple decision.

Walking is *much* safer than running. It pampers your musculoskeletal system, where running can jiggle and bounce you to chiropractic disaster. Because the walker lands with much less force than does the runner, you put your ankle, knee, and back at far less risk.

Adherents of walking as exercise run the gamut of emotions with respect to how much they like walking. Many come to consider it a pleasure that they would pursue even if it had no health benefits. But we would be less than honest if we did not admit that there are some people who simply hate exercise of any sort and figure that God wouldn't have given us labor-saving devices had he not wanted us to use them.

We won't kid you by telling you that there is some magic way to make exercise a task you love if you are one of these people. However, there are *many* things you can do to make the road to health less wearisome to travel. The specific nature of these varies with the individual.

Walkers who are not among those enamored of the scenes of nature that greet the walker find their Walkmans as indispensable as their walking shoes. Some go so far as to program specific tapes for each day's walk in an effort to forget, as far as possible, that they are walking. If you are one of these, stop feeling guilty and start recording. Your body doesn't care whether you *like* walking, only that you do it.

If you dislike music almost as much as walking, avail yourself of the immense library of books on tape. A number of companies now put unabridged works on tapes that last from six to nine hours. Two such tapes a month and in a year you'll be not only healthy but well read.

If all this sounds a bit lonely for you, go in the other direction to make walking more pleasurable: join a walkers' club. Such clubs can be found almost everywhere, and you'll be amazed how much faster the time passes when you're having a good conversation, rather than counting how many steps you've taken.

Whatever your method, be sure to vary your route. Variety is

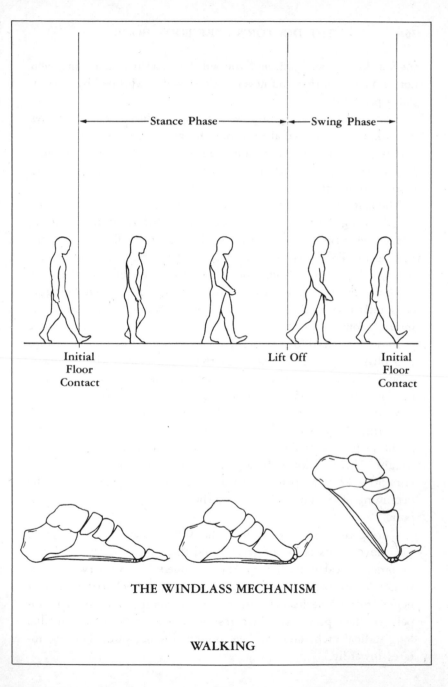

Stance Phase — Swing Phase

Initial
Floor
Contact

Lift Off

Initial
Floor
Contact

THE WINDLASS MECHANISM

WALKING

the antidote to boredom, and you will be amazed at the things you notice on a walk that you never noticed as you whipped by at sixty miles per hour.

Let us assume that by now we have so convinced you of the joys of walking that you've already put the book down and given it a try. It might increase your enjoyment to learn a bit about the role gait plays in your newfound activity. The issue is considerably more complex than you might suspect.

The gait cycle is a series of events, expressed in percentages, that occur during a single step. It starts with the right foot making contact with the ground and ends when the right foot makes contact again. For every second, indeed every fraction of a second, during this cycle—from the time the heel first strikes the ground—the joint motions and muscle positions are changing so constantly that even the largest computer can·only approximate the interrelationships.

In order to make this all comprehensible, we divide the gait into two phases, the stance phase and the swing phase. The former is about 65 percent of the cycle and the latter is—bet you've figured this out already—35 percent. (These figures can vary by about 5 percent, but don't worry about that—we don't.)

During the stance phase there is an initial period, amounting to about 12 percent of the entire cycle, in which the foot bears double weight. This is followed by a period of single-limb support, which lasts from 12 to 50 percent of the cycle. From this point until the beginning of the phase there is another period of double-limb support.

During the first 15 percent of the walking cycle the body must slow down at its center of gravity and then immediately accelerate in order to carry itself over the extended leg. Otherwise there would be no forward motion. At the point of heel strike the foot begins to become loaded with the body weight. For this to happen, the foot pronates, which results in a lowering of the medial longitudinal arch, and the heel bone turns outward. The leg rotates inwardly.

During pronation the joints of the foot loosen so that the foot can adjust and take the measure of the surface beneath and absorb the inevitable shock. At this point there is little muscle activity.

Muscle activity begins in earnest during the next stage. While the foot is still supporting less than the entire weight of the body, the leg muscles and the intrinsic foot muscles go into action. The heel begins to invert and the foot begins to supinate. At this point there is external rotation of the leg, the forefoot is fixed to the floor with the heel in inversion, and the foot becomes a rigid structure.

During about half of the walking cycle the load on the weight-bearing foot exceeds that of the body weight by about 25 percent. The foot begins to plantar-flex, the arch becomes rigid, and the heel lifts off the ground. The plantar fascia shortens and the toes begin to flex, creating a "windlass action" that elevates the arch. This all energizes propulsion that is followed by the swing phase, which makes up the final 35 percent of the gait cycle. When the heel strikes the ground again, the cycle is completed.

At the midpoint of the stance phase of the gait cycle, the foot should be in neutral position. Pronation is normal and to be expected in the initial-contact phase, but it should not be present in the final, propulsion phase. Similarly supination is normal during the latter stage but not the initial one.

The hallmarks of the normal gait are involvement of the pelvis, the swing limb, the stance limb, the thorax, and the upper limbs. The pelvic motion is upward, forward, and to the side of the stance limb. The pelvis rotates with the swing-phase limb, tilting to the side of the swinging limb.

Consequently the swing limb shortens by flexion of the hip and knee, lifting the foot off the ground and permitting inward rotation of the foot, tibia, and femur. The stance limb, on the other hand, allows inward and outward rotation, flexion, and extension of the hip, knee, ankle, and toes. The thorax rotates in the direction opposite the pelvis, while the upper limbs exhibit a swinging motion on the opposite side of the swing limb.

The normal gait is the background against which abnormalities of gait are judged. The trained observer can gain insight into an individual's gait and the normal gait.

To be sure, there is a range of motions considered normal. These usually concern tempo and rhythm and, above all, they are symmetrical. Note how often you have assessed a person's mental state from his walk. The depressed person slouches and shuffles, while the happy person bounces along.

Likewise, physical conditions can be indicated by gait. There are four general groups of pathological gait, each associated with specific forms of pain, deformities, paralysis, and lack of coordination.

Antalgic gaits are those in which the abnormality of gait alleviates pain. The specific antalgic gait will depend on where the pain is located, but the most familiar is that associated with avoidance of back or abdominal pain. When this is the situation, the gait is guarded, with slow, careful steps and reduced movement of pelvis and thorax. Subtleties of gait permit further identification of the area of problem: in lower-back pain the vertebral column might deviate forward or backward, while lateral pain forces one to favor the sound side.

If the problem is sciatica, on the other hand, the step is shortened on the involved side. Hip, knee, or foot pain will cause a slight flexion and a shortened stance phase on the involved side. In general, pathological conditions tend to alter as the individual attempts to shift the body mass to the sound side.

Joint problems, such as ankylosis or a contracture of the soft tissues, can cause a shortening of a limb and a resulting short-leg limp. Involvement of the hip joint will keep the knee in flexion during the stance phase and, on some occasions, the trunk will bend forward in a bowing motion.

Perhaps the easiest of the less-dramatic abnormal gaits to identify is that caused by the stiff knee. As the foot clears the ground, the limb will swing outward and forward in a semicircular movement technically known as a hemicircular gait. Patients exhibiting this gait will sometimes raise themselves on the toes of the opposite side, causing a vaulting gait.

Foot deformities cause gait abnormalities that are easily recognizable. Some examples are walking on one or the other part of the foot, an unusual deviation in the angle of the foot placement as in in-toeing and out-toeing gaits, an unusual deviation in the width of base as an abducted or crossing-over gait, and an exaggerated outward rotation of the leg during the stance phase.

Virtually any deformity, whether inherited or congenital, will alter the gait. A short-leg limp is, not surprisingly, characterized by a drop of the body upon stance on the shorter limb. In cases where the affected limb is only two inches or less shorter than the normal limb, there may be only a slight pelvic drop without foot compensation. However, a greater disparity often forces the individual to hold the foot in an equinus position, which manifests itself in a tiptoeing gait on one side. Sometimes the disparity between legs is so great that even this doesn't suffice, and it is necessary for the person to shorten the longer leg by bending it at the knee and hip.

The precise nature of a paralytic gait is determined by the muscles involved in the paralysis. No two cases are exactly alike because the site and severity of the paralysis will affect the type and form of the compensatory gait. In many cases the paralytic gait is named for the muscle whose paralysis is causing it: quadriceps gait, gastro-soleus gait, triceps paralysis, gluteus medius paralysis, and ankle dorsiflexor paralysis are typical names. The last of these is characterized by a high knee raise, foot drop, and loud slap of the foot against the floor.

Gait disturbances resulting from central nervous system disorders are referred to as dyskinesia. Many of these are familiar accompaniments of well-known and serious diseases. Cerebral palsy often engenders a scissor gait with knock knees and a spastic equinus position of the foot. Multiple sclerosis manifests itself in a rigid-legged spastic gait. A person with Parkinson's disease will often have a gait characterized by hurried, short steps. People with advanced syphilis will often exhibit an ataxic gait in which there is uncertain placement of the foot, inappropriate effort, and a failure to maintain a rhythmic pace. Certain cerebral lesions can cause a gait similar to that found in one who is intoxicated.

While the elderly are vulnerable to many of the diseases that cause abnormality, such abnormalities are more often caused by combinations of the problems that affect the aged. Most familiar, perhaps, is the senile gait disorder that leads old men to develop a flexed-position walk of wide-spaced, small steps. Women affected by the same disorder tend toward a narrow-based, waddling gait. The elderly of both sexes tend to fear falling and, indeed, have a tendency to fall backward.

In addition various medications often prescribed for the elderly can cause gait abnormalities even in people who would not otherwise have them. The benzodiazepines can cause an intoxication characterized by disorientation, sedation, or agitation and a progressive deterioration of the gait. Antidepressants can cause a Parkinson-like gait, while salicylate intoxication can produce an imbalance that can alter the gait. All of the threats to the elderly are magnified by the brittleness of elderly bones and the potential for problems affecting the bones to take away the old person's independence.

Fortunately appropriate treatment is increasingly capable of forestalling the bone diseases that disturb the gait.

Running for Your Life
(or Running from It?):
Running

Millions of people are running for recreation and fitness. Some have a very casual approach to the sport; however, many people take running very seriously and it is an important part of their lives. It has all the advantages associated with walking and the disadvantage of being a high-impact sport. The dynamic loading on the human musculoskeletal system is 3.6 times greater during running than during walking. The chance of injury to the runner is considerably greater than to a person engaged in a walking program.

Running is marvelous for the respiratory system; it really does make you feel good. It definitely improves your general health and it may prolong your life. (The jury is still out on this, but the evidence seems to be favoring the view that running can increase longevity.) The down side is that unlike, say, rowing, which causes very few difficulties for one without back problems, running can be to your feet what Attila was to the peaceful countryside.

Exacerbating the threats to your feet inherent in running is the unfortunate fact that running seems to become an obsessive pursuit too easily for too many people. It has been well established that six to ten miles a week will do all that running can do for you; hundreds of thousands of people do ten or more times this for reasons not explicable in terms of their rationalizations.

If you run fifty miles a week because you enjoy it, fine. But if you think you're doing your body and feet a favor, forget it. Running has only the time factor favoring it over walking, and for this it introduces a host of possible high-impact traumas.

There are three basic types of running: In order of distance they are the sprint, the middle-distance, and the long-distance. The line separating the sprint from the middle-distance is blurred because the definition of the sprint is blurred. Some define the sprint as a race in which per-yard speed is constantly increasing. However, strictly speaking, this would exclude the hundred-yard dash. Runners slow down after about sixty yards, and when it looks like the winner is pulling away from the pack, he is really just slowing down less slowly than his opponents. Others define the sprint as a race in which you run as fast as you can throughout, while still others define it as a race in which there is little strategy (that is, little laying back, and so forth). The important point is that a sprint makes few demands on the aerobic systems you wish to improve. (However, "wind sprints"—a series of sprints—can be of major aerobic significance.)

Middle-distance races are usually considered to be those from about half a mile to two miles, with long-distance now including races as long as a hundred miles.

For our purposes the important differences among the distances concern the gait. Each distance has its preferred gait.

The sprinter's gait is one in which the foot strike is almost solely on the forefoot and the body is leaning forward more than would be the case at the other distances. In middle-distance running the heel and forefoot share the honor of striking the ground, while the long-distance gait more closely resembles a speeded-up version of the walking gait.

Perhaps the most important difference between the running and walking gaits is the absence of any double-limb support in the former. All three types of running have periods of "floating" in which both feet are off the ground. To see this in action, simply start walking and increase to a run; notice how the float phase develops as you speed up. The more you increase your speed, the more you decrease the time your foot touches the ground. A stance phase of six-tenths of a second in walking is reduced to a fifth of a second when you run. As the stance time decreases, the demands on your foot are increased and can become greater than three times body weight. For a two-hundred-pounder this means the muscles must endure over six hundred pounds of force through a range of motions for which walking has not prepared it.

Even the most sedentary among us have experienced the reality that the range of joint motion in the lower extremities is dramatically extended when we run. The surprise is not that so many people encounter injuries, but that there is anyone who doesn't.

But as we have hinted, it is not the basic act of running but the obsessive need to run at times when rest is indicated that fosters most injuries. The overwhelming enthusiasm that many serious runners have for the sport is probably the root cause of most injuries associated with the sport. The desire to run farther, faster, and for longer periods of time leads to the most common injuries found in the sport, overuse syndromes of one type or another. These types of injuries respond well to a decrease in the training schedule but present an extremely difficult problem to the practicing clinician, as it is very difficult to get a runner to slow down or cut down on distance or speed. Every podiatrist will tell you that his most wasted efforts are his long warnings to inveterate runners to take it easy, warnings the podiatrist knows will go unheeded.

It is a peculiarity of running injuries that one injury almost guarantees a secondary injury. Overcompensation (where rest is indicated) to protect an injured leg multiplies the probabilities that the second leg will pay a price. A great deal of pronation in a hypermobile foot will invite subluxation of the patella. In this case, as in others, the *proper* antidote (in this case an arch support) can solve the primary problem without introducing a secondary problem.

Pain in the knee is the most common complaint among distance runners. Often this reflects a transrotational problem of the patella. When the runner has an unusually high arch, the pain can be substantial because the foot lacks even an average ability to absorb shock. Runners with normal feet sometimes manage to mimic the high-arched-foot runner by wearing shoes with inadequate absorption capacities.

The list of similar problems is endless. Running on a curved indoor track can cause pain in the calf and knee resulting from internal rotation of the leg and incorrect push-off. An externally rotated right foot can result in lateral patellar pain.

Sometimes a secondary problem suggests the solution to a primary problem, and this solution solves both problems. Sciatica, for example, can be secondary to weak abdominal muscles. Build up the abdominals and the sciatica disappears.

The role played by running surfaces in producing injuries is difficult to overstate. Whatever their other virtues, the new synthetic surfaces are far less friendly to the runner's foot than were the old grass and cinder tracks.

The very thing that enables these surfaces to increase performance, the increased traction they permit, is the thing responsible for increased numbers of injuries. Increased traction means that the foot has less room to slide and pivot, and the hard surface beneath magnifies the shock wave that greets the foot. You might not know it, but your joints do, as this can lead to damage and destructive processes in the joints of the lower extremity. The harder the surface, the more rapid and severe the joint destruction.

Even the competitive racer should do nearly all his training on grass or cinder and save the synthetic surface for the actual race (and just enough training runs to acclimate to the track).

The orthotic that is a help to the noncompetitive runner is a requirement for the racer. Orthotics are possibly the single most efficient way to reduce stress on the musculoskeletal system by engineering the insole to absorb the impact that would otherwise be forced on the foot itself.

Shinsplints, pain and tenderness over the anterior aspect of the lower leg at the level of the anterior compartment, is a common complaint among runners. As common as this problem is, we are still not certain of its cause. The most likely culprits are training errors like too-quick increase of training frequency or duration, resuming training at the level where the runner left off before a long layoff, changing from natural to artificial surface, overstriding, and wearing improper or improperly fitting footgear.

Anatomical factors associated with shinsplints include flat foot, leg-length inequality, high arches, and muscular imbalance and inflexibility. Physiological changes such as a decrease in bone density owing to hormonal changes in amenorrheic women athletes can contribute greatly to this problem.

A study in South Africa found that subjects reporting shin soreness had significantly greater range of subtalar and talar joint motion and significantly lower percentages of calcium intake coupled with an increase in training intensity just before injury. This is a relatively minor problem that gradually improves with conditioning.

Stress fractures of the tibia can sometimes mimic shinsplints, but it takes diagnosis by bone scan to tell that this is the case. Rest and *gradual* return to activity usually alleviate the problem, but in more difficult cases taping, arch supports, and special footwear may be required.

More involved and more incapacitating than shinsplints is the chronic compartment syndrome. To understand this condition, a bit of anatomy is required.

There are four compartments within the leg: the anterior, lateral, superficial posterior, and deep posterior. The former contains the foot dorsiflexors and inverters and the toe extensors. The lateral compartment contains the primary foot plantar flexors, while the last contains the foot inverters, additional secondary plantar flexors, and the toe flexors.

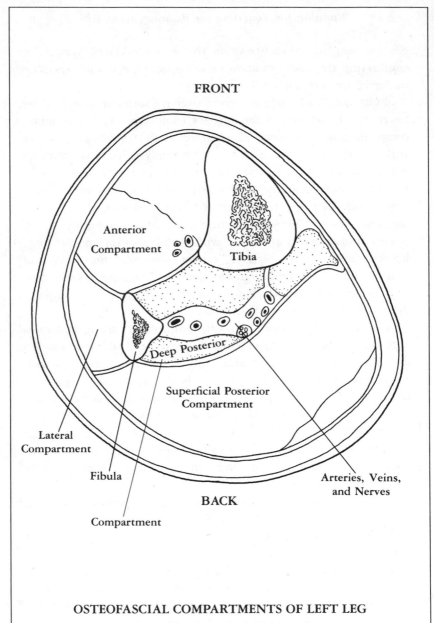

FRONT

Anterior
Compartment

Tibia

Deep Posterior

Superficial Posterior
Compartment

Lateral
Compartment

Fibula

Arteries, Veins,
and Nerves

BACK

Compartment

OSTEOFASCIAL COMPARTMENTS OF LEFT LEG
CROSS-SECTION BELOW KNEE

The most common compartment syndromes affecting the runner are those involving the anterior, anterolateral, and deep posteriors. Like other compartment-syndrome conditions, these are the result of an increased tissue-fluid pressure in a closed osteofascial space, a situation that compromises the circulation to the nerves and muscles within the space and engenders hemorrhage or edematous fluid accumulation within the closed compartment of the extremity. If nothing is done to begin decompression, nerve and muscle damage will ensue.

A chronic compartment syndrome is often the result of exercise that caused a rise in intercompartmental pressure sufficient to compromise small vessels and introduce secondary ischemia and pain. (Normal intercompartmental pressure is 0–8 millimeters mercury; with exercise, levels rise above 50.)

After a given number of miles the runner will complain of pain in the anterolateral compartment and a secondary numbness on the top of the foot. While the symptoms will subside after a period of rest, diagnosis can be made immediately from a pain disproportionate to the clinical situation, paraesthesia, burning associated with nerve distribution within the compartment, a tightness within the compartment, pain on passive stretching of the muscles, and a latent weakness of the involved muscles. The pain is described as a deep, throbbing feeling of pressure and is sufficient to cause the runner to cease exercise at the inception of the pain. Interestingly, there is no alteration of the pedal pulsations. They are easily felt by the doctor. It is the microvasculature that is closed down from the pressure.

Treatment consists of resting the involved area, nonsteroidal anti-inflammatories, and a subsequent decrease in running mileage. It is far from unknown for surgical decompression to be required. As soon as healing permits, both active and passive exercises are begun in order to preclude extensive stiffness.

It is the rare runner who has not suffered heel pain. While such pain can be caused by an inferior (bottom) or posterior (back) calcaneal spur on the heel bone, it is more frequently the result of plantar fasciitis. The pain will often radiate into the arch area when this is the case. This is because the plantar fascia—a thick, fibrous band of connective tissue on the plantar surface that runs forward to the metatarsal heads as it fans out—supports the longitudinal arch and assists push-off during running.

Not surprisingly plantar fasciitis is an overuse injury that follows sudden increases in mileage, frequency of running, or speed. Running on hard or unyielding surfaces will aggravate this condition, particularly in feet that tend to pronate. If there is a burning pain in the heel or arch, it is the result of increased strain on the plantar fascia caused by the downward movement of the longitudinal arch.

Treatment consists, as usual, of a relative rest, avoidance of hill running, and decreases in mileage and frequency. Ice applications can be helpful and anti-inflammatories can reduce swelling and pain. If the problem is chronic, correction of pronation and a shortened Achilles tendon is indicated. These are accomplished with an orthotic device that keeps the subaltar joint in a neutral position. Sometimes the mere addition of an elastic heel lift one-eighth of an inch high will do the job.

If an important race is near, an adhesive strapping of the longitudinal arch may be necessary. Commercially available heel cups may reduce the pain. Exercises to increase flexibility of the Achilles tendon, stretching twice a day on a heel-cord box, and stretching with the heels straight will all increase the flexibility of the soleus muscle. Overall condition can be maintained by alternative activities such as cycling. Surgery is saved for the most recalcitrant cases and is usually avoidable.

While it is not usually the culprit, stress fracture must always be considered when a runner complains of heel pain. X rays are ineffective for diagnosis; a nuclear bone scan (which will reveal increased uptake of radioactivity in the heel) must be utilized.

Compression syndromes of branches of the posterior tibial nerve in the heel cause a burning pain that may require surgery.

Runner's toe is caused by repeated trauma of the nail of the first toe, which results in blood clot under the nail (a subungual hematoma) with characteristic blue discoloration of the nail. This occurs most often when the runner wears shoes that are too tight in order to increase traction. During deceleration this forces the foot into the toe box and traumatizes the first nail. Proper fit and toe padding eliminate the problem.

Toe problems can also occur when otherwise normal digits are longer than the other toes. The longer toe receives a disproportionate amount of trauma and shows its unhappiness by turning blue. This condition is usually benign and rarely requires treatment.

In addition, of course, runners can be affected by all of the maladies that affect nonrunners. These can play havoc with a training schedule.

Some authorities consider running barefoot perfectly safe, and the world-famous Zola Budd chooses to run barefoot. For the average runner, however, there are two very good reasons for wearing running shoes: protection from everyday environmental hazards such as nails, broken glass, and the like; and the impossibility of using corrective orthotics if you are going barefoot.

Orthotics came into the mainstream of American life as runners increasingly realized their value. To use just one example of their abilities, orthotics can control arch problems and transfer pressure points. Soft, pliable orthotics made of felt, foam, or similar inexpensive materials can be fabricated by the athlete himself if he is the slightest bit handy. These can be worn on a temporary or long-term basis, if they help, and can be renewed or refashioned as the situation warrants.

A semirigid or semiflexible orthotic must be made by a podiatrist. These are made of heat-sensitive materials immersed in hot water or baked in an oven and are relatively inexpensive. Their purpose is to keep the foot in a neutral position.

A rigid orthotic is a somewhat more involved and expensive procedure, but one that has brought relief to thousands who had previously suffered debilitating and painful conditions. A mold is made of the patient's foot and the orthotic is made from that mold, much like false teeth. Posts or bars are added to increase rigidity and force the foot into a neutral position. Rigid orthotics will last an extremely long time if correctly cared for.

Correct choice of the orthotic is dependent on correct diagnosis of the problem. Identification of the precise type, place, and depth of pain aids this process. Many questions will be asked, and it behooves the individual to think carefully when answering. When did the pain begin? Is it associated with a specific motion? Did the patient skimp on warm-up or stretching? Is there inflammation? Did it worsen upon a change in training methods, distances, or speed? Was any new factor introduced? A new surface? New shoes? Damage to a shoe? Wear patterns?

Sometimes the experienced runner can solve a problem by asking such questions and attending to the problem in a way that the answers suggest (though this is not the case of course if rigid orthotics are indicated). As a rule heat will increase pain, swelling, and inflammation in an acute injury. Cold compresses, mild compression, and elevation of the injured part will often relieve mild injuries.

But if discomfort continues, professional advice must be sought. In the long run this is usually the most cost-effective and least painful way to treat your feet well.

Many of the principles that apply to the selection of walking shoes also apply when buying a running shoe. Because there are ten running shoes for each walking shoe, you may at first be overwhelmed by the range of choice that faces you. Don't be. A few simple questions can suffice to eliminate most types and models.

Do your old shoes demonstrate any unusual wear patterns? Do you have any specific chronic aches or pains in your feet? Do you have a history of problems related to running? What kinds of surfaces do you most often run on? Are you overweight? These questions alone will serve to reduce the number of potential shoes to a manageable few.

Begin by finding a store that has a large selection and a good reputation. No salesman has ever told a buyer that the shoe for him was one that his store didn't sell. Stick to well-known brands and be suspicious if the salesman seems to be pushing one you never heard of. As a rule, good shoes are relatively expensive; unfortunately so are some bad shoes. However, if you buy a shoe of a respected manufacturer that costs a bit above the average for that manufacturer's line, you will probably be buying a good shoe. This is not a good place to look to save money.

As is the case with walking shoes, you must look for heel durability, adequate cushioning of the ball of the foot, and rearfoot stability. Examine the insides of the shoe carefully for any irregularity that might cause irritation.

Fit is crucial, so try the shoes in the afternoon, when your foot has expanded to its largest size. Try on both shoes and wear the socks you will run with. Make certain your toes do not touch the front of the shoe and use the same test as for walking shoes: There should be a thumb's width between your toes and the end of the shoe. You are looking for comfort and stability, so make sure the heel fits snugly and comfortably.

When you try on the shoes, tie them snugly. There should be a thumb's distance between the lace holes on either side of the shoe.

If you already wear orthotics, you must use them when trying on new shoes. The shoe that feels fine without orthotics will not feel fine with them, nor can it render the orthotics unnecessary. When you try the shoes, remove the insoles.

There is no such thing as a shoe that is right for everyone. The model that your friend finds the route to heaven may be your path to hell.

There are, however, shoes that are wrong for all runners. Do *not* substitute tennis shoes for running shoes. Tennis is different from running. The tennis shoe lacks the cushioning in both the heel and the forefoot a runner needs for protection from shock. The tennis shoe is constructed primarily to withstand the rigors of lateral movement, and the runner moves forward, not laterally. (You probably knew that.)

A reminder: If your running shoes get wet, do not force-dry

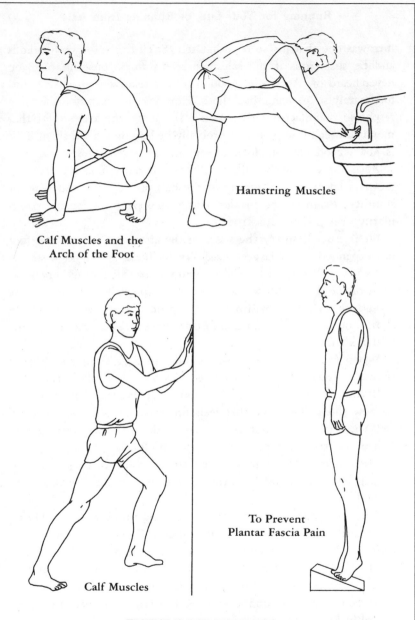

Calf Muscles and the
Arch of the Foot

Hamstring Muscles

Calf Muscles

To Prevent
Plantar Fascia Pain

FLEXIBILITY EXERCISES

them. Allow them to dry naturally overnight. If they are made of leather, saddle-soap and polish them. A well-cared-for running shoe is a runner's best friend.

Once the shoe issue is settled, and before you hit the trail, you might try a few simple exercises that can increase flexibility and lessen the likelihood of injury. For the calf muscles and arch of the foot, kneel with your toes curled under your feet. Slowly sit back on your heels until you feel the tension in the bottom of your feet. Hold this position for thirty seconds and repeat three to five times. *Never bounce.*

Another calf muscle exercise involves placing one leg two steps away from the wall. Carefully lean toward the wall, supporting yourself with your arms. Bend one leg and keep the other straight. Keep both heels on the floor and slowly move your hips until you feel tension on the calf of the straightened leg. Again: NEVER BOUNCE.

To increase the flexibility of the hamstring muscles in the backs of the thighs, place your right foot on an object lower than your hips (such as a car bumper). Carefully bend forward at the waist until you feel tension on the hamstrings. Hold for thirty seconds and relax. Repeat three to five times, slightly increasing the pressure each time. Now do the left side. No bouncing!

Finally, if you are wondering why we never discuss "jogging," rest assured that jogging is, for our purposes, the same thing as running.

The Toes of Toddlers:
The Child's Foot

You probably didn't notice it at the time, having more important things to think about, but the story of your feet began in the fourth week of your embryonic life.

The limb buds that were to eventually become your arms, legs, hands, and feet contained the ectoderm that represented the seminal forms of skin, hair, sebaceous glands, and mesoderm, which, in turn, generated bones, muscles, tendons, and ligaments. Nerves and blood vessels are not generated by the bud material, but tunnel through as continuations of the nerves and vessels of the trunk of the body.

The lower extremity develops in a proximal-to-distal (near-to-far) direction. Thus the thigh develops, then the leg, and finally the foot. The growth of the foot follows the same pattern, with the rearfoot developing before the forefoot.

After the fifth week the foot begins slowly to take shape and become recognizable. You can make out, as a tiny prominence, that which will become the big toe. At this point the foot is positioned in such a way that the plantar surface faces the head and middle of the body. As it develops, however, it rotates in a more medial direction.

At the nine-week point that differentiates the embryonic from the fetal periods, the soles of the feet face each other, often even making contact. Bones have not yet ossified, and the ankle joint shows no sign of the angulation that will later distinguish it. But as development continues, the feet slowly turn downward and away from each other, continuing their transformation into the appendages that will later cause us so much trouble.

Some of the congenital troubles are easily recognized at birth. It does not take years of training to notice polydactyly, the presence of extra digits. These extra toes can be on the side of the first toe (preaxial), on the side of the little toe (postaxial), or in the center, duplicating one of the middle toes.

Polydactyly is most common among females and blacks and is a dominant hereditary trait. Treatment, as you no doubt guessed, consists of surgical excision of the extra digit.

Syndactyly (webbing of the toes) and *microdactyly* (small toes) rarely require medical treatment, though some patients opt for surgery for cosmetic reasons. The same is true of cleft foot (lobster-claw foot), a deformity in which the second, third, and fourth metatarsal and phalanges are deficient.

Congenital hallux varus presents as a medial angulation of the great toe. It afflicts the sexes equally, and in about a third of the cases both feet are affected. This is one of the cases in which conservative measures nearly always fail. The same is true of various types of hammer toes, mallet toes, and curly mallet flexed toes.

In some cases a malformation is best treated within hours of birth. An example of this is a condition medically known as talipes equinovarus, but familiarly referred to as clubfoot. Clubfoot is a complicated deformity composed of three key elements. The "club" condition results from the ankle being in equinus, the subaltar joint in varus, and, likewise, the mid and forefoot in varus.

Though usually inadequate, nonsurgical techniques are attempted first. The feet are manipulated to a position of maximum correction and held there by tape or cast. This is repeated every few days or weeks and then once a week for a few weeks. If these manipulation and immobilization techniques fail, as they usually do, a surgical release of the Achilles tendon, ankle capsules, subaltar joints, and joint capsules must be initiated. Surgery performed at the age of two or three months is nearly always successful. However, in a significant number of cases the involved foot can have excess soft tissue on the lateral side, and a permanent decrease in calf size is not uncommon.

A *congenital vertical talus,* or rocker-bottom foot, is characterized by a malposition of the navicular on the head of the talus. These are bones in the rear part of the foot. There is a vertical placement of the talus and a dislocation of the subaltar joint.

Diagnosis in such cases is relatively simple: The sole of the foot is convex, with a distinct rocker-bottom appearance and a prominence of the head of the talus on the medial and plantar aspect. The heel is in equinus and valgus, and the forefoot is dorsiflexed and abducted. Deep creases can be noted on the dorsolateral aspect of the foot anterior and inferior to the lateral malleolus. The foot is rigid even when not weight bearing and markedly pronated. It is easy to recognize children with this condition; they exhibit a very awkward gait and poor balance. They walk with feet outturned, rolling into valgus. The psychological effects cover a surprising range. Some children are embarrassed by the malformation, while others seem virtually unaffected in other than the obvious physical ways.

This congenital deformity can occur alone or in conjunction with other congenital deformities, such as contracture of joints (arthrogyposis) or protrusion of the spinal cord through a defect in the vertebral canal (myelomeningocele). As is the case with clubfoot, this abnormality must be treated immediately if treatment is to be maximally effective. Again as with clubfoot, manipulation and tape or cast immobilization is worth trying. Even if not sufficiently successful, these procedures facilitate surgical procedures if any of a number of surgical procedures prove necessary.

It is the unfortunate fact, one that is crucial to remember, that any visible birth effect can indicate a defect that is not visible. Extreme dorsiflexed first toes and rocker-bottom foot are associated with cardiovascular and renal abnormalities.

Congenital constriction band syndrome manifests itself in bands of concentric rings that may be shallow or deep. This condition is not hereditary. It appears as a mechanical entrapment of the parts involved. In the foot it is the great toe that is most frequently involved. The distinction between congenital and hereditary is important to understand.

Hereditary conditions are passed down through the genes. Congenital conditions result from an embryonic or fetal event affecting a previously normal embryo or fetus. The reason for the confusion is the fact that, particularly before the days of amniocentesis, each was first noticed at birth.

In any case congenital constriction band syndrome is primarily a male affliction and thought to develop in the fifth or sixth embryonic week. This syndrome is highly associated with clubfoot.

When shallow, the ringlike bands tend to involve only the skin and subcutaneous layers. However, when they penetrate more deeply, the rings compromise the venous system and lymphatic return. The result is edema and enlargement of the area distal to the band. In the worst cases the limb may undergo spontaneous amputation in utero. This can sometimes be avoided if noticed sufficiently early for several stages of surgery to be performed.

At birth the foot of the infant is longer proportional to the body than is the case with the older child. The joints are so supple that it is possible to dorsiflex the foot until it touches the anterior aspect of the leg; likewise the foot can be plantar-flexed to become parallel to the tibia, the leg bone.

The toddler's foot is also somewhat more chubby and wider than that of an older child. Because there is fat in the area of the medial longitudinal arch, parents often believe, incorrectly, that their baby has flat feet. By the time the child is five, this sole fat has disappeared and the arch has a normal appearance.

These realities can be seen most clearly in sole prints. That of the two-year-old seems to represent the flattest of possible feet. Sole prints of the same child three years later demonstrate that there was never anything to worry about.

In some cases, of course, children really do have flat feet. Often this need not be treated, and indeed a careful biomechanical evaluation is mandatory before any treatment is prescribed or implemented.

If weight bearing results in collapse of the arch, treatment is recommended. The purpose of the treatment is to maintain the foot in a neutral position. Orthotics enable the bones to grow in as normal a position as possible. Exercises strengthen and stretch the muscles to conform to the increasingly normal formation of the bone. In less serious cases arch supports glued in the shoe may suffice.

There is a simple test that enables parents to get some indication of whether their child has an arch problem. Called the great-toe extension test, this consists of simply having the child stand upright and looking forward while putting full weight on his foot. The parent then dorsiflexes the great toe without any help from the child.

If the child's foot is normal, the dorsiflexion will cause the arch to rise, the foot to supinate, and the tibia to rotate externally. Failure of the test suggests functional abnormalities of the foot.

An abnormally high medial longitudinal arch is referred to as a pes cavus. A contracture of the plantar surface and abnormalities of the skeletal architecture prohibits normal flattening of the arch and maintains the heel in a varus position. Contracture of the soft tissue that is supposed to support the longitudinal arch worsens the condition. Specifically the spring and short plantar ligaments combine with alteration of the plantar fascia to create this deformity.

People with this condition often complain of pain in the soles of the feet, unusual fatigue, calluses, and areas of irritation under the metatarsal heads—all of which make finding comfortable shoes nearly impossible.

There are a number of possible causes of pes cavus. Problems of the nervous system (specifically Charcot-Marie-Tooth disease), poliomyelitis, and spinocerebellar degeneration can all be responsible.

In mild cases nonsurgical therapeutic techniques can successfully solve the problem. Orthotics, metatarsal bars applied to the shoes, and a reduction of painful lesions are often sufficient in the case of young adults. If the condition is congenital, manipulation and casting are usually required. For the infant, application of a Denis-Browne bar to the shoe is often sufficient to rectify the problem.

A Denis-Browne bar is a device that is affixed to the shoes for the purpose of rotating the foot to an external position, usually of about forty-five degrees. Despite their looking a bit like an item of medieval torture, Denis-Browne bars, which are worn only during periods of sleep, are painless and very effective. After a day or so the child pays no attention to the device, though the parents can often present a problem.

Complementing the application of the Denis-Browne device is a correction of the shoe consisting of an outside sole wedge (lateral) and an inside heel wedge (medial) of about one-eighth to one-quarter of an inch. These are applied to the exterior of the sole and heel of the shoe in an effort to attain eversion of the forefoot.

If, however, the device is not enough to solve the problem, one of many case-specific surgical procedures almost invariably gets the job done.

While there is still some question as to its nature, osteochondritis, also known as osteochondrosis, is thought to be an avascular necrosis (lack of blood supply) of the growing center of the bones of the foot. The primary cause seems to be trauma, resulting either from a single major episode or from a series of minor shocks to the foot.

As you might guess, the endless activity of the child, particularly running and jumping, can easily cause a trauma to the weight-bearing parts of the foot, and these can interrupt the supply of blood to the bone. Often there is local swelling that leads the child to limp, but even when this is not the case, palpation points the investigator to the problem. X rays, which expose a "moth-eaten" appearance of the involved centers, verify the presence of osteochondrosis.

When osteochondrosis attacks the navicular bone, the syndrome, first described in 1908, is known as Köhler's disease. Köhler's disease affects six boys for every girl, usually makes its appearance between the ages of three and eight, and is found in both feet only 30 percent of the time.

Typically the patient complains of a pronounced pain in the navicular area and can be observed to walk with a pronounced limp. Initial X rays reveal a condensation and increased density, and a posttreatment follow-up of several X rays will show quite clearly the fragmentation and repair.

Treatment for Köhler's disease is conservative. In cases where pain is severe, immobilization by a short cast is helpful. Unna boots and flexible castings with tape are often indicated. Treatment is symptomatic and takes six to eight weeks, after which the child is usually comfortable and able to proceed without pain.

Because the navicular bone is at the apex of the medial longitudinal arch, it will be affected by many other problems besetting the foot. For this reason it is necessary that any preexisting pronation be corrected. Otherwise the probability of recurrence is high. Orthotics are pressed into service to accomplish this. In less-severe cases Köhler's disease passes unnoticed and uncommented upon— until it is betrayed by adult X rays, which show an undersized and abnormally shaped navicular.

Osteochondrosis of the calcaneus is referred to as Sever's disease. Characterized by a pain in the heel bone, it is also an avascular necrosis of the growing center of the heel (the epiphysis). The pain of Sever's disease, while not extreme under quiet conditions, increases rapidly with activity, and the active Sever's patient usually walks with an antalgic gait. When palpated, the posterior heel exhibits severe pain, particularly if the practitioner squeezes from medial to lateral.

As with Köhler's, Sever's usually attacks boys, though somewhat older boys. Like most of the disorders we discuss, occurrence in the teen years is far from rare. As with Köhler's, X rays provide a definite diagnosis, and conservative treatment is usually successful. Because this malady involves a shortening of the Achilles tendon, stretching exercises are most helpful.

Freiberg's infraction is an avascular necrosis of the head of the second metatarsal. First described in 1914 by A. M. Freiberg and then again in 1920 by A. Köhler, this is often referred to as Köhler's disease number 2. Unusual in that it is more commonly found in females, it can occur in the third, fourth, or fifth metatarsal head as well as in the second, but the latter is the most common site. Following onset, usually in adolescence, pain is limited to the areas that actually bear weight. Palpation magnifies such pain.

Once X rays verify the expected flattening of the metatarsal head, crutches will sometimes be used to ease immobilization. Subsequent use of orthotics with a metatarsal raise can be useful if long-term therapy is indicated. If untreated until adulthood, Freiberg's may require surgery.

Osteochondrosis of the talus involves the medial dome of the talus. It is like the afflictions we have just discussed, save for the fact that it is the anterior aspect of the ankle joint that responds to palpation.

Beneath the head of the first metatarsal bone are two pea-shaped bones called the sesamoids. A traumatic event, such as a fall on the ball of the foot, can engender an osteochondrosis that is discoverable by palpation of the sesamoids directly. Even before palpation, however, the problem is suggested by an inability to walk on tiptoe without great pain. Pads placed along the plantar aspect of the first metatarsal will protect the area from trauma when the patient is walking. Crutches, followed by orthotics, are usually the therapeutic path indicated.

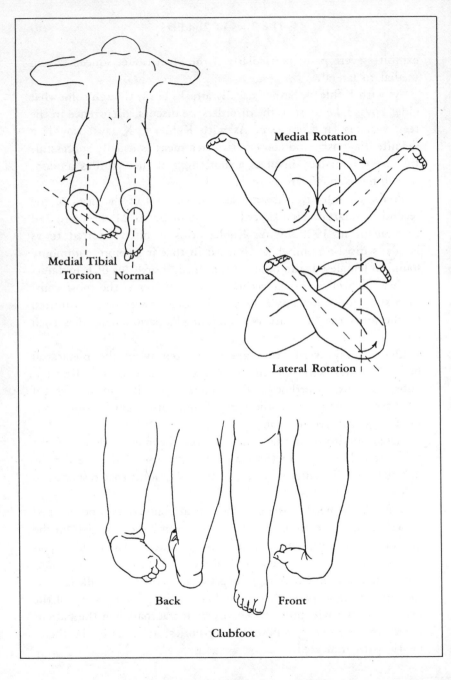

Medial Rotation

Medial Tibial
Torsion   Normal

Lateral Rotation

Back   Front

Clubfoot

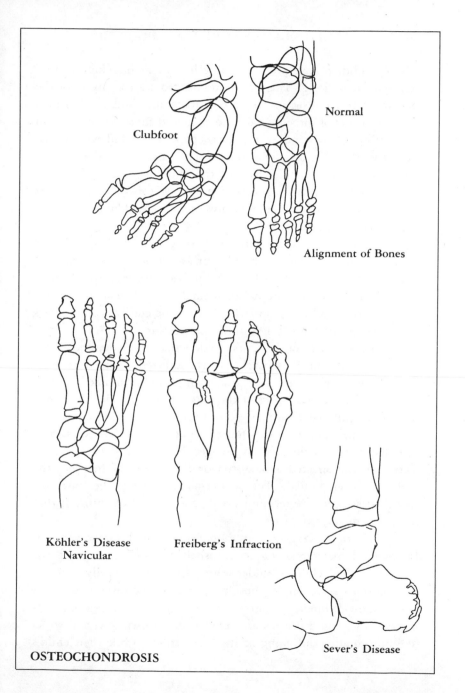

Clubfoot

Normal

Alignment of Bones

Köhler's Disease
Navicular

Freiberg's Infraction

Sever's Disease

OSTEOCHONDROSIS

Many children have problems of gait such as intoeing, outtoeing, and toe walking. The former results from a turning in of the forepart of the foot (as in the case of metatarsal adductus). Additional elements of intoeing vary, so the child must be observed in both walking and standing modes (both barefoot and with shoes) for a correct diagnosis to be made. The position of the knee is noted under these conditions and the child is then made to lie prone with knees bent to ninety degrees. At this point in the examination of the sole of the foot any metatarsal adductus problem can be spotted easily.

Here is why. If you draw an imaginary line, it should, under normal conditions, line up the plantar aspect of the foot, leg, and thigh. When these fail to line up, it becomes easy to diagnose internal tibial torsion, internal or medial femoral torsion, or anteversion of the hip by appropriately having the child keep the knees flexed and moving his feet inward and outward.

When mild cases of metatarsus adductus are recognized early, conservative treatment is nearly always sufficient. Passive stretching of the baby's forefoot at diapering time, combined with a stroking of the lateral aspect of the foot, often precludes the necessity of complicated treatment. However, if the condition is still present as the infant enters its fourth month, it will be necessary to introduce serial castings, changed weekly. Each cast extends correction of the affected area until, over a period of months, the problem is eradicated. For a period following the castings, straight-last shoes are recommended as a method of ensuring that the problem stays resolved.

The situation is considerably more serious for children over two. Pronounced metatarsus adductus usually means surgery for the post-infant. For children under eight, surgery is usually required only on soft tissue, but for those over eight, bone surgery is likely.

It is most common for parents to come into the office complaining that their child is awkward, trips over his own feet, and walks like he's coming and going at the same time. While their child's awkwardness is understandably upsetting, the parents are more often than not unnecessarily worried. Often their child has a hip anteversion, also known as an internal medial femoral torsion, that causes the gait problem, which parents usually notice when the child is beginning his third year. In fact the problems caused by this syndrome, if bothersome at all, are primarily cosmetic and amenable to conservative treatment. Often it becomes apparent as the child ages that there is nothing worth worrying about, and by the time the child is six, the issue is usually forgotten.

The quasi-reverse of internal torsion, outtoeing, is usually, though not always, self-correcting. This external lateral femoral torsion has its root in a congenital tight Achilles tendon or, on some occasions, in poor initial walking habits. It also occurs in milder forms of cerebral palsy, but the primary condition is usually identified before the minor foot problem manifests. When habit is responsible for the genesis, games encouraging the child to walk on his heels is all that is required. If the problem is congenital and serious, surgery may be indicated to lengthen the Achilles tendon.

For all children, from those who enter the world with normal feet to those with the most serious abnormalities we have discussed in this chapter, correct choice of shoes is crucial.

Shoes serve two primary functions: warmth and protection from sharp and rough objects. Despite the surprising number of people who believe the contrary, shoes are not necessary for the child to learn to walk. After all, there have been many societies in which people walked and ran with grace and skill without ever having seen a shoe.

But shoes are, in modern, industrial society a necessity and must conform to health needs if they are not to harm the child. For the child learning to walk, softness is mandatory so that the child can learn to sense the contours of the ground. The shoes should not have heels, which can catch on carpets and random objects.

When buying their child new shoes parents should allow for the growth that inevitably follows immediately and should make certain that the uppers are sufficiently soft and flexible to prevent rubbing. Hightops offer some added stability, but their greatest virtue is their resistance to the child's attempts to kick them off.

In general it will be necessary to change the child's shoes every three months. Signs of redness and irritation around the toes are a sure sign that shoes are too small. Children between six and nine are in the period of life in which the foot grows the fastest and must be checked even more often than usual.

The understandable desire to avoid the cost of new shoes leads many parents to give the child hand-me-down shoes. Don't do it. Shoes should conform to the child's foot, not force his foot to conform to the foot of another.

School-age children should have several pairs of shoes, and extreme styles should be avoided. It is probably impossible to get a little boy to forgo cowboy boots altogether, but at least they should be worn sparingly. Teenagers will gravitate to whichever currently fasionable shoe is worst for them, and there's nothing you can do about it. Common sense can go a long way in the area of footgear.

How Can Something So Small
Hurt So Much?:
The Infected Foot

Feet are funny. Most of the time. Until, that is, even the slightest of infections stops the laughter. The poor human foot is hopelessly misused and neglected the world over.

Anyone who has ever suffered from even the smallest blister has learned how much agony can come from pressure on a tiny spot. Often the vehicle for this pain is pressure; a blister filled with the residue of infection (pus) presses outward in all directions. When you step on the blister, causing inward pressure, the pain can be shocking. And we're only talking about a blister.

Fortunately this pain is our friend. (Yes, really.) People don't ignore pain, so they get the pain-causing problem attended to before the problem becomes life-threatening.

In most cases. Some sources of chronic, rather than acute, pain override the alarm system by paralyzing or killing the nerves that serve as pain messengers. Leprosy is one of the more gruesome, and increasingly rare, examples of this. As we will see, pain in the foot can be a signal of not only a foot problem but of a systemic problem that will kill if not arrested. Diabetes, for example, is often discovered by its effects on the foot.

Infections of the foot are divided into three parts: bacterial infections of soft tissue and bone, superficial fungus infection, and deep infection associated with chronic systemic disease. The last of these differs from the first two in that its usual entree into the localized area is not through a break in the skin, but in the blood coming from a previously infected part of the body.

Most of the time foot infection is the story of bad guys slipping through an opening in our first line of defense, the skin. Our skin is not there just to prevent our insides from being on the outside. Skin is our separation from all those things in the environment that threaten our insides. It doesn't do much good against lions and tigers (that's why we have brains), but it is a miraculous defense against the infinitely more numerous threats that we can't even see, the bacteria.

Usually the skin works fine. But when a cut or rip in the skin opens a path, a million bacteria will notice and immediately set up housekeeping.

Because the foot would otherwise be so vulnerable to infection (and other problems), nature has provided us with thicker skin on the bottom of the foot than anywhere else. This skin differs from that on most of the rest of the body in that it is without follicles and therefore hairless, and consists of two layers, the epidermis and the dermis. The epidermis, which can be viewed as essentially a four-layer stratum, is approximately 1.4 mm thick, about half the thickness of the dermis.

The dermis is composed of two layers, the papillary (which makes contact with the epidermis) and the deep layer called the reticular layer.

Farther down there is a subcutaneous layer of connective tissue comprised mostly of adipose tissue that carries the blood vessels and nerves. This, termed the superficial fascia, is the arena for much foot infection. Superficial-fascial spaces include web spaces (which correspond to the webbings between the toes), interdigital spaces, and heel spaces. The deep-plantar spaces are divided into the medial, the central, and the lateral.

When any of these spaces become infected and filled with pus, the swelling and the pain the swelling causes can be awful. Moreover it is often the case that the port of entry is relatively far removed from the site of infection. For example a tiny crack at the level of one of the web spaces can infect a superficial-plantar space.

The infection with which most of us are most familiar is the *blister*. The simple blister, which affects only the epidermis, is filled with a clear liquid that lifts the epidermis and gives the familiar blister bubble. This, in and of itself, is technically not an infection. However if the irritation continues, as it is likely to if one is hiking or playing tennis, it becomes very likely that infection will ensue.

If the abrasion is unattended and the epidermis and dermis continue to break down, we can expect the development of an ulcer that exposes the subcutaneous tissue. This tissue did not evolve to be an infection fighter (that is the job of the epidermis and dermis). Thus it provides fertile areas for bacteria to flourish. If this is permitted to continue, major soft-tissue structures, such as the tendons, become involved. Finally infection of the bone (*osteomyelitis*) threatens the foot and is very difficult to treat.

A similar chain of events can be caused by injuries due to mechanical violence ("wounds") such as crushing, punctures, or tearing away of the skin. In all such cases the threat of infection is magnified by contamination by dirt, chemical substances, and other foreign bodies. When this occurs, the wound must be debrided very carefully.

A *puncture wound* presents an even greater potential for serious damage. A nail, needle, or other sharp object can provide a direct path to the deep structures for anaerobic organisms (ones requiring no oxygen) capable of causing serious illness. Most of you are familiar with the best-known of such illnesses, *Clostridium tetanus*. In many such cases surgery is necessary to permit drainage and a direct assault on the infection.

In "degloving" accidents, when large amounts of skin are lost, the threat of infection is very great, and extensive anti-infection measures must be taken.

Bacterial infections of the soft tissue of the foot are many and varied, as are their causes. Here we will survey typical examples of the different types.

Cellulitis is an infection of the dermis usually caused by a staphylococcus organism. While its usual point of entry is a cut in the skin, this organism is also capable of entering through the hair follicles of the dorsal surface of the foot. Cure is a virtual certainty if the patient can be persuaded to complete a program of antibiotic medication, complete rest, and elevation of the foot.

Lymphangitis, an infection of the lymphatic channels and the lymph nodes, makes its appearance known with a sudden onset of chills, fever, and localized pain. Within twelve hours the lymphatic channels are marked by bright red lines, and the lymph node proximal to the channel becomes swollen and painful. If these are not treated immediately, septicemia can develop. For the patient with lymphangitis, bed rest is an absolute necessity. Antibiotics in many of these cases are administered by injection and/or intravenous drip.

A *Whitlow,* often referred to as a *felon,* is an infection of the pulp space at the distal phalanx of the toe. Its most identifiable symptom is a severe and throbbing pain. Pus collects in the tip and bottom of the toe, causing considerable pressure and pain. This threatens to erode the bone at the tip of the toe, causing osteomyelitis. It is often necessary to surgically open the area to permit drainage.

Acute infectious tensonyvitis is a bacterial infection of the tendon sheath. It is usually a result of the spreading of infection from an adjacent area that was accidentally lacerated or contaminated in a puncture-type wound. Once the practitioner has followed the anatomical development in the tendons of the affliction, he can determine the extent of the infection and can initiate the required, usually aggressive, treatment.

There is only one normally occurring anatomic bursa in the foot, the retrocalcaneal bursa, which is found just behind the heel. Other bursa, called adventitious bursa, are built by the body to protect underlying bony structures. Both sorts of bursa can become infected. A familiar example of an adventitious bursa is that associated with a bunion deformity.

We have a number of times referred to *osteomyelitis,* a bone infection. Usually carried to the bone by the blood, osteomyelitis is the work of *Staphylococcus aureus* and is always to be taken seriously. It is a threat whenever one suffers a compound fracture and it often requires aggressive antibiotic therapy and surgical drainage.

If the acute stage of osteomyelitis is not treated promptly and correctly, the development of chronic osteomyelitis is exceedingly likely. While the chronic variety is less painful than the acute, it can cause destruction of soft tissue and bone. As this occurs, drainage sites, exhibiting bits of dead bone, appear through the sinus tracts. At this point surgery is very often required.

There is a special type of osteomyelitis in which a localized intramedullary abscess is walled off within the bone. Called a *Brodie's abscess,* this commonly occurs in males, usually at the distal aspect of the tibia at the ankle joint. Symptoms of Brodie's often last for a number of years and then subside.

To this point we have been discussing infections caused by pus-producing organisms, the most common of these being staphylococcus and streptococcus. Under a microscope these are easily distinguishable. The former appears as spheres in clusters, a grape-like look, while the latter tend to group in a straight line.

There are, however, chronic infections of the foot that are not associated with pus-producing organisms. For example it sometimes happens that, for reasons unknown, bone density in a given area increases without abscess or pus formation. Known as *Garre's osteomyelitis,* this is treated by surgically excising the dense bone.

In other cases there is infection but not pus. *Tubercular infections,* caused by the rod-shaped mycobacterium tuberculosis, can have a secondary effect on the feet. You don't tend to think of tuberculosis in terms of the feet, but it is not uncommon for the disease to manifest itself in a severely arthritic ankle. It reaches this destination through the bloodstream. Setting up camp in the soft tissue in and around the joints, it eventually comes to a temporary rest in the articular cartilage. It then invades the cortex of the bone and forms nodular cold abscesses. These subsequently drain through sinus tracts of the skin.

Treatment in such cases is difficult. Antibiotic treatment must be aggressively pursued for at least eight months. If the ankle joint is involved, there will be a narrowing of the joint space and an erosion of the articular cartilage, causing joint pain and stiffness. The foot gradually goes into downward position and loses its ability to bear weight.

If the disease is caught at the soft-tissue stage, complete healing and return to normal function can be expected. However, once the articular surface becomes involved, there is little hope of a restoration of normal joint functioning. The same is true of involvement of the talus that forms the mortis of the ankle joint and the lower end of the tibia. Solitary lesions in other bones of the foot, while they do occur, are rare. This is an unrelentingly destructive disease that must be fought with all the powerful weapons at our disposal.

The foot is not the first organ that comes to mind when we think of syphilis, but this does not render it immune to the ravages of this disease. *Syphilis* is caused by the *Treponema pallidum,* an organism of spiral shape and voracious appetite. It is usually acquired sexually but can be transmitted from an infected mother to a fetus.

Before the advent of modern antibiotics, syphilis was one of the leading causes of death and insanity and the leading cause of joint destruction. Jean-Martin Charcot did the first of his groundbreaking studies of *Charcot's joint* not on the diabetics with whom he is usually associated but with syphilitics.

Joint damage from syphilis is often found in the knee, but ankle involvement is not rare. In both cases pain and disability are to be expected. Toe involvement (*dactylitis*) is a manifestation of the con-

genital form of syphilis in which the toes become swollen and spin-
dle-shaped.

Diagnosis should be prompt in the case of syphilis and other
sexually transmitted diseases (such as a gonococcal infection) borne
to the foot by the blood; this usually affects both feet at the same
level, attacks the soft tissue first, and ultimately destroys bone.

There are many *mycotic* (fungus) *infections* of the feet, the most
simple of which is the familiar, and easily cured, *athlete's foot*. Far
more serious are such fungi as those that cause *Madura foot*. Like
athlete's foot, these enter through fissures in the foot or cracks in
the heel. They can also be borne by the blood. The disease is
especially prevalent in the Madura region of southern India, hence
its name.

The fungus (or, occasionally, a false fungus) enters through the
sole of the foot and forms nodules under the subcutaneous layer of
the skin. These nodules enlarge and break down, forming multiple
sinuses. If not stopped at this point, the soft tissues and, ultimately, the joints will be involved. While there is a surprising
absence of pain, the foot can become enlarged and grossly deformed.

The false fungus to which we referred is the actinomyces bovis.
It is a filamentous organism that resembles a fungus but is more
closely related to a bacterium. It is found in the United States and
develops in the same manner as the Madura fungus.

Most commonly affecting the proximal and middle phalanges of
the toes of young males, *sarcoidosis* is a chronic infectious disease
marked by granulatomous lesions of the bones of the foot. There is
swelling, pain, low-grade fever, and redness. In extreme cases the
toe can become mutilated.

We do not know how *leprosy,* also known as Hansen's disease, is
transmitted. It is thought to be caused by the organism
Mycobacterium leprae. Contrary to popular belief, it is the slowest-
proceeding of all diseases. Slow or not, it is capable of bone damage and often generates arthritic ankle leprous lesions. These cause
a neuropathy and insensitive foot, and can cause foot drop resulting

from peroneal nerve damage. Treatment is complicated and very long-term.

Yaws is a contagious, infectious disease caused by a spirochete similar to that causing syphilis. Unlike syphilis, yaws is not a sexual malady. It is usually acquired in childhood and transmitted directly through broken skin. It makes its initial appearance as a multiple raspberrylike granulomatous bump on the skin and is subsequently characterized by an inflammation of the periosteum, the tough, fibrous membrane that surrounds the bone. It is in the tertiary and final stage of the disease that the foot becomes significantly involved. Irregular, deep ulcerations of the soles become deeply fissured. The metatarsal and phalangeal bones of the feet become thick and show signs of destruction. The treatment is what one would expect: antibiotics and attention to the local fissures.

There are a number of *parasitic infestations,* of which that caused by the guinea worm is typical. The infected larvae enters the body in contaminated drinking water and matures within the unsuspecting human host. The adult female worm negotiates the openings in the subcutaneous tissue and causes a blister that can be quite large. When the foot makes contact with water, the worm works its way out through the skin to discharge her eggs. Treatment consists of taking oral medications and the physical extraction of the worm from the foot.

Finally, *gas gangrene* can be a late, and potentially fatal, stage of a number of diseases that prepare the way for the clostridium bacteria. The clostridium is an anaerobic organism that grows deep in a wound. Since it does not need oxygen, this limitation on most bacteria does not even slow down the clostridium. Gangrene is an ever-present danger in cases of crush injuries. When it strikes, it does so with alarming speed and extreme toxicity. Antibiotics are of limited value. However, because this organism flourishes in dead tissue, surgical removal of any such tissue can halt the spread in its tracks. If caught early enough, such surgery is minor. Waiting too long can mean amputation or death.

This Little Piggy
Got Stepped On:
The Injured Foot (and Ankle)

The foot is the bumper of the body. If there is trouble in the area, your foot is likely to get to it first.

And there are so many kinds of trouble that can be too much for your feet. Needles, gunshots, large objects dropped from high places, broken glass, splinters—my, oh my, the list is endless. These dangers differ in many ways. But from your foot's point of view they have one thing in common: They hurt.

Burns are one of the more common trauma-inducing events affecting the foot, and often these have causes other than fire. Many a podiatrist must weekly treat burns from chemicals applied by overzealous patients who tried inadvisable acid preparations in attempts at self-treatment. Radiation, which can cause ulceration requiring skin grafts, and electrical shock can likewise do serious damage to dermal and subdermal tissue.

In the latter case, the injury is directly proportional to the duration and force of the current. Alternating current can cause deep tissue damage that is easy to miss on a cursory examination by a

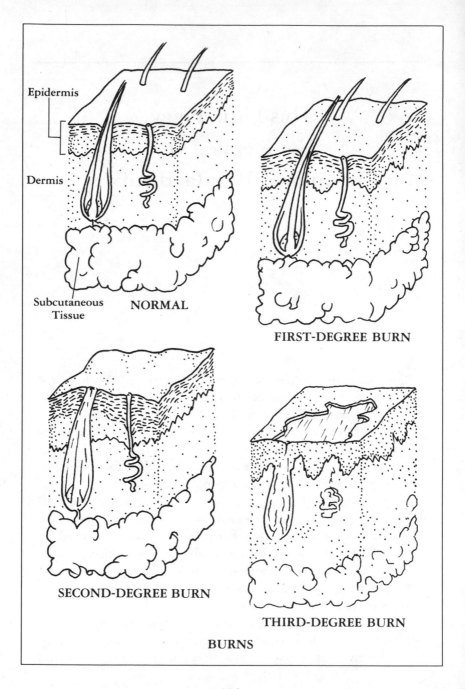

Epidermis

Dermis

Subcutaneous Tissue

NORMAL

FIRST-DEGREE BURN

SECOND-DEGREE BURN

THIRD-DEGREE BURN

BURNS

podiatrist. Such damage requires a thorough debriding of the deep tissue.

Burns from hot liquid are common and usually the result of an accident in the home, rather than work. When such a burn on a child is bilateral and symmetrical, child abuse must be considered a possible cause.

Burns are categorized by their degree of damage as first-, second-, or third-degree. Unlike murder, the *higher* the degree, the greater the seriousness.

First-degree burns are characterized by redness and dryness of the skin, with an absence of blistering. A mild sunburn is a first-degree burn.

Second-degree burns involve a more pronounced redness, swelling, moistness, some loss of sensation, and blister formation. This is often the result of scalding but can be caused by a bad sunburn on the feet, an event remembered forever by one who has experienced it.

A *third-degree* burn involves the epidermis, dermis, and underlying tissue. It almost always brings with it a loss of sensation.

Treatment of a burn is determined by the degree and type of the burn and can run from local application of a topical medication and dressing to surgical debridement and full-thickness skin grafts. Contracture and scarring caused by burns will sometimes necessitate reconstructive surgery and braces for support.

The first stage of treatment, however, is the determination of the seriousness of the burn. American Burn Association guidelines categorize a burn as "minor" if it involves less than 10 percent of the body (5 percent in children), is less than 2 percent full thickness (both layers of skin), and does not involve primary areas of the body. ("Primary areas" are the face, perineum, hands, and—what interests us here—feet.) Foot burns, in other words, must be taken *very* seriously.

Initially a burn must be treated with cold compresses or cold water. If ice water is used, care must be taken to prevent frostbite. NEVER apply butter or grease. This old wives' remedy merely forces the doctor to clear out the material, causing a loss of valuable time and making further injury likely. Butter and grease are not only unsterile, they are also likely to promote bacterial proliferation leading to infection. Such infection, often caused by streptococcus organisms, can require hospitalization. Fortunately these bacteria are vulnerable to penicillin and can be controlled in a hospital setting.

When a burn is superficial and there is no necrotic tissue, treatment can be limited to a mild emollient cream to limit edema and pain. A second-degree burn must be cleansed and the blisters opened and drained with a sterile needle. The skin over the blister is left intact to prevent infection and to limit the pain of exposed raw skin. (This route should be followed even with a normal blister due to walking.) A third-degree burn forms a tough, adherent eschar that should be left intact until normal separation occurs.

Burns of the feet are always potentially dangerous and must always be treated with the utmost seriousness. They must be treated promptly and correctly if long-term disability is to be avoided.

A *crush injury* to the toe or foot involves all the tissues of the affected area and must be considered serious and dangerous until professionally proven otherwise. This entails professional cleansing, removal of all weight bearing by the affected area, compression dressing, and elevation. The injured area is closely watched until it is clear that the possibility of involvement of additional tissues has passed.

The tendons are particularly susceptible to trauma. Tendon injury can run from a simple tenosynovitis to a complete rupture of the tendon. *Tenosynovitis* is an inflammation of the sheath surrounding the tendon. All tendons of the foot, save the Achilles tendon, have such a sheath.

Virtually everyone who has played a too-vigorous game of tennis or run that one mile too many has experienced a tenosynovitis at one time or another. More serious is a direct blow to the tendon, an injury that is likely to generate a hemorrhagic tenosynovitis with blood flow into the tendon sheath. This is more difficult to treat than is the simple tenosynovitis.

When the foot is cut open during an injury, laceration of the tendon is always a possibility. Early treatment is vital, as torn and cut tendons often respond well to primary suture repair. This is particularly the case when the large Achilles tendon (which inserts into the back of the heel) is ruptured; delay can result in a lifelong, drastic alteration of the gait.

To evaluate an Achilles-tendon injury, the podiatrist must thoroughly palpate the gastrocnemius muscle in the back of the leg through its entire length. A test known as the Thompson squeeze test can help determine whether there is a partial or complete tear of the tendon.

The Thompson test is performed in this manner: The patient sits on the examination table with his legs hanging down. The podiatrist squeezes the large gastrocnemius muscle in the back of the leg. This will cause an uninjured foot to plantar-flex. The injured foot, on the other hand, will demonstrate little or no response, and the examiner can determine the degree of injury from the response or lack of same. A patient with a partial tear will walk with a flat-footed shuffle on the injured side.

All the bones of the foot are subject to fracture, but here we can discuss only *fractures* of the major bones. Fractures of this sort are a major problem in heavy industry: they result in the loss of one working day per month per twenty workers.

The most commonly fractured tarsal bone (the large bones of the rearfoot, not the metatarsals or toes) is the calcaneus or heel bone. Ninety percent of such injuries happen to men younger than forty-five and involved in industrial occupations. Economically such an injury can be disastrous, as it can incapacitate the patient for up to three years and partially incapacitate him for up to five. These types of fractures are classified by the part of the bone that is broken and the resulting disability that follows this classification.

Treatment varies with the type of fracture and can consist of immobilization and supportive measures, on the one hand, or internal fixation with pins, screws, and wires, on the other.

Fractures of the talus, the bone forming the mortis of the ankle, are relatively uncommon, but can cause serious difficulties and disability when they do occur. Fractures of the midfoot (navicular, cuneiform, and cuboid) are also uncommon, and these cause less disability and require less treatment when they do occur.

Fractures of the metatarsal bones occur frequently and are often overlooked, thereby causing a delay in treatment. There are five metatarsal bones in each foot, and studies have shown that the fifth metatarsal, the one nearest the outside of the foot, is the most easily fractured. This is because the base can be easily torn away as a secondary result of a severe inversion sprain of the ankle. The least commonly fractured metatarsal bone is the fourth.

Treatment varies as a function of the specific injury. If it is an open fracture (the bone breaking through the skin), treatment will be different from that required for a closed fracture. Displacement and nondisplacement will also play a role in determining treatment. In all cases aggressive and comprehensive treatment will usually lessen long-term disability.

Fractures of the bones of the toes (of which there are fourteen in each foot!) are by far the most common fractures of the foot. Nearly everyone has smacked his or her little toe into a bedpost, and many have earned a "broken toe" as a result.

Fractures of the first toe are extremely common and can involve long-term periods of disability. Whichever the toe, treatment will be determined by location and severity. Fractures of the fifth toe, for example, can often be treated by merely taping it to the adjacent toe, which acts as a splint.

When a bone is weakened by cyst, tumor, or disease, a spontaneous fracture can result. In World War II soldiers occasionally developed fractures from the pounding a foot takes during a march even when there was no single traumatic blow. Treatment of these sorts of fractures is case-specific.

The most common types of acute trauma encountered by the podiatrist are those to the ankle joint. Each year four million people suffer ankle injuries and pay over $2 billion to have them treated.

Because these injuries are so common, a short recap of the relevant anatomy is in order.

The ankle is essentially a hinge. It is formed by the tibia (above and medially), the fibula laterally, and the talus below the tibia and between the malleoli. The talus fits into a mortise formed by the tibia and fibula. Medially the distal tibia ends as a short, thick projection called the medial malleolus.

On the lateral side the distal end of the fibula becomes the lateral malleolus, which is lower than the medial malleolus. The body of the talus lies between the medial and lateral malleoli and articulates with the tibia above, the medial and lateral malleoli on each side, and the calcaneus below. The head of the talus, which runs slightly downward and inward, articulates with the navicular. The top surface of the talus is wider anteriorly than posteriorly. The medial aspect of the joint is strengthened by the deltoid ligament, a very strong triangular band. The lateral aspect of the joint is strengthened by the fibular collateral ligament, which, in turn, is comprised of three separate bands. There are thirteen tendons that cross the ankle joint, the largest being the Achilles tendon.

There is no pure up-and-down movement of the joint, because plantar flexion is accompanied by heel inversion and forefoot adduction, and dorsiflexion is associated with heel eversion and forefoot abduction.

There are six basic mechanics of ankle injury: inversion, eversion, external rotation, dorsiflexion, plantar flexion, and axial loading. It is the mechanism of an injury that furnishes the best indication of which of the supporting ligaments might be injured.

A *strain* is a stretching without tearing of the muscles, tendons, or ligaments. Strains are extremely common and often occur from simple overuse, without any noticeable twisting of the ankle. Such strains nearly always respond well to rest, ice packs, and, if necessary, such support as an elastic bandage. If you are physically active, you can assume that you'll encounter a strain every so often.

Ankle *sprains* are more involved, and more capable of causing disability, than are strains. Inversion sprains are the most common, followed by eversion injuries involving the medial side of the ankle. (See also the section on sprains in the following chapter.) These often occur in athletes at a moment when a pronated foot is planted firmly and the lower leg is struck laterally.

These forms of ankle sprain are many and varied, and it is beyond the scope of this book to examine each in detail. Suffice it to say that any but the most minor sprain will require professional attention. However, you can begin by checking the circulation. Squeeze the toenail or pulp of the great toe and check for capillary refill. A slowness of the refill process will alert you to the possibility that blood vessels have been compromised.

Neurological evaluation is more difficult. Obvious nerve damage can be ascertained by pinpoint or two-point evaluation. Palpitation can indicate the area of most damage, and gently moving the foot through its range of motion can often tell the mechanism of the injury.

The anterior-drawer test is a simple test that can effectively identify the degree of injury. The tibia is held steady with one hand. With the thumb of the other hand held over the talus and the second and third fingers behind the calcaneus, attempt to move the talus forward and backward on the ankle mortis. Compare the two feet. Any difference in draw between the affected and unaffected ankles—particularly greater excursion on the injured side—suggest a rupture of the anterior talofibular ligament.

Ankle injuries are classified according to grade. A grade-one injury has a partial tear of the anterior talofibular ligament. Grade two entails this plus a partial tear of the calcaneofibular ligament. A grade-three injury implies complete disruption of both of these.

There are alternative methods for classifying ankle injuries, but this is the most comprehensible and therefore the most widely used.

Grade-one and grade-two sprains are usually treated nonsurgically. Grade three usually presents a surgical situation.

Whatever the grade of the injury, initial treatment is of crucial importance in heading off further damage. Ice packs applied immediately to the affected area are, as we have seen, very effective in controlling pain and swelling. Elevation is usually indicated. Many professionals continue to use elastic bandages for support and control of swelling, but the truth is that they are of limited value. Ice, elevation, and nonsteroidal anti-inflammatories usually accomplish as much as can be accomplished at the early stages of an injury.

As soon as possible, active range-of-motion exercises should be begun with an emphasis on strengthening the muscles on the outside of the lower leg, and stretching the muscles at the back of the lower leg. You must be careful if you attempt passive range-of-motion exercises; your partner cannot sense your pain as instantaneously as you can and can force the injured area too far too fast. Unna boots, which are soft-type casts, are often advised for a week or so following the first forty-eight hours.

For patients who suffer chronic sprains and ankle instabilities, rehabilitation exercises can be very helpful. A useful exercise for strengthening the anterior compartment consists of looping a rope through a five- or ten-pound weight (a paint can filled with the appropriate amount of weight is fine) and draping the rope over the forefoot as you sit on a table or desk. Fifty repetitions of dorsiflexion and plantar flexion with the foot in neutral position, internal rotation, and external rotation are sufficient. Other helpful exercises are discussed in the chapter on the dancer's foot.

Above all, never simply neglect the simple sprain and hope it will go away. It won't, and neglect can lead to weak ankles and arthritic complications from altered gait.

Strapping or taping of the ankle region is a tried-and-true approach that has been used for many years, particularly by athletes. Useful as these may be, however, it is important to remember that they are only part of a rehabilitation program.

Unlike the shoulder, which precludes taping because of its great range of motion, the ankle lends itself to strapping modalities. But the taping must be done by someone else if it is to be effective; self-taping procedures are almost always ineffective.

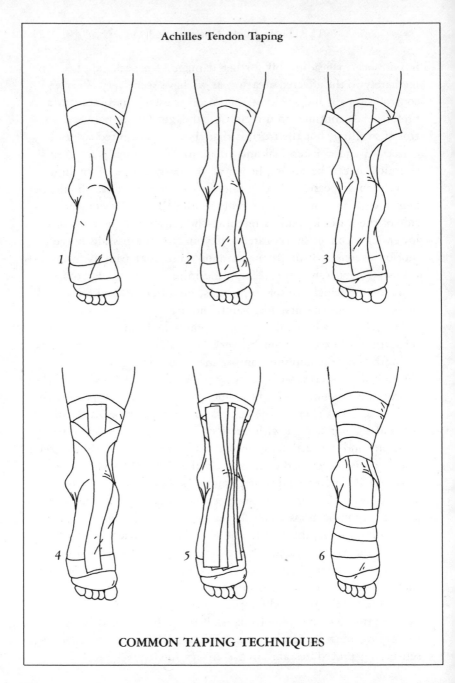

COMMON TAPING TECHNIQUES

Basketweave

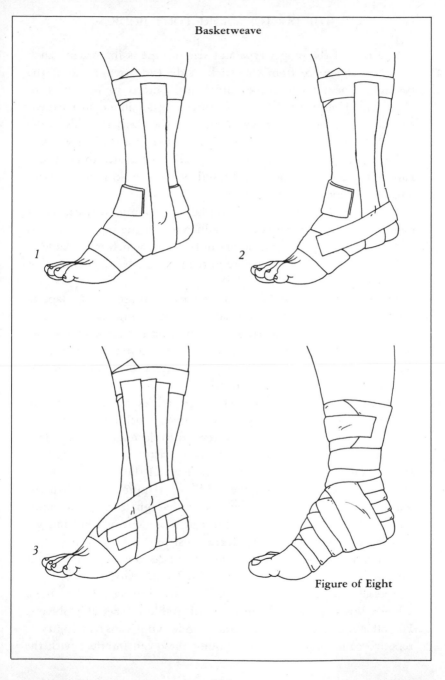

1

2

3

Figure of Eight

Selection of the proper type and size of tape is important. Look for good adherence from the sticky side and strength from the backing. The tape must be sufficiently porous to permit it to "breathe." Unfortunately these features are not found in inexpensive tapes. Elastic tapes are excellent, but the elasticity adds to the cost. Whatever the tape, it should be stored in a cold, dry place.

Be sure to attend to the care of the skin of the area to be taped. Failure to do so will lead to a breakdown of the skin and you will have to abandon tape altogether.

Remove all hair from the skin, either by shaving or by the use of depilatories. (This permits better adherence of the tape and avoids irritation.) Apply a bit of tincture of benzoin, which is available in a convenient aerosol form, before putting on the bandage to further guarantee adhesion.

Do not give in to the inevitable tendency to use enough tape to mummify the body. It is the quality of the taping, not the quantity of the tape, that matters. Incorrect or excessive taping can introduce circulation problems, which is the last thing you need. Remember, the goal is to restrict movement by duplicating the anatomical structures externally.

Elastic wraps as substitutes for tape trades avoidance of skin breakdown for support. They are, of course, much easier to remove and do provide considerable compression to decrease swelling. It is best to use a good-quality, three-inch elastic bandage, working from distal to proximal. Begin at the level of the metatarsal heads and work backward toward the ankle, overlapping about half the width of the bandage as you go. A figure-eight turn at the ankle will increase support. Use gentle but firm pressure as you bandage, keeping the ankle at a ninety-degree position. If you are treating a common inversion-type ankle injury, place the foot into slight eversion in order to support the injured ligaments.

Special attention should be paid to the injuries of the young athlete, whose growing bodies are vulnerable to special problems. For all athletes the most common underlying cause of injury is repetitive microtrauma. In the young these can interfere with the sporadic growth of muscles, ligaments, and tendons. When these are in growth stages, they increase in tightness and decrease in flexibility, greatly enhancing the potential for injury. The skeletal immaturity of the young athlete renders him susceptible to microtrauma in the growth cartilage located at the epiphyseal plates, the joint surfaces, and the insertion sites of major muscles and tendons. The foot and ankle are especially vulnerable.

Similarly the articular surfaces of young knees and ankles are threatened by shear forces to a far greater extent than are the mature knees and ankles of older athletes. Young runners, during the pubertal growth spurt, develop tight, strong quadriceps and gastrocnemius-soleus muscles and tight, weak hamstrings. For these youngsters, stretching exercises to increase flexibility and joint motion are a necessary preventative to injury.

Overzealous parents and coaches, and overintensive sports camps, are responsible for many athletic injuries. An uninvolved individual should investigate the demands made by parents, coaches, and camps to avoid the athlete's being placed in a dangerous situation.

While all athletes should be concerned with nutrition, the requirement is especially important for one whose body has not reached maturity. High fat, high sugar, and junk foods simply cannot provide the vitamins and minerals necessary for an intensive training regime. Likewise the avoidance of good foods as well as bad by amenorrheic athletes doubles the probability of stress fractures made possible by low bone density. Good nutrition and the appropriate vitamin and mineral supplements can reduce this probability.

Proper footgear is a barrier against injury. Follow the guidelines given throughout this book and remember to wear shoes specific to the sport you are playing.

It is always advisable to check the young athlete for anatomical malalignments, patellar problems, knock-knees, bowlegs, and flat feet. All of them predispose one to injuries caused by the repetitive stress of athletics.

When an injury does occur, the RICE regimen proves a tried-and-true treatment. RICE equals Rest, Ice, Compression, and Elevation. Rest equals refraining from all aggravating activity. Ice equals ice (or cold) applied to the area to lessen pain and swelling and to slow metabolic activity in injured tissue. Compression equals the use of an elastic bandage. Elevation equals keeping the injured part higher than the heart for the first twenty-four hours after the event.

RICE is a valuable technique for treating the stress fractures that are particularly common among adolescent athletes. It is helpful for tendinitis and the common inflammation at the sites of tendon insertions known as apophysitis.

Adolescents are prone to sports-related overuse injuries of the lower extremity at the hip, pelvis, knee, ankle, and foot. If not recognized early, stress fractures of the proximal end of the femur can have devastating consequences. The gymnast is particularly prone to this threat.

Overuse injuries are as varied as microtrauma in the knees caused by running up and down bleacher stairs and the calcaneal apophysitis that attacks runners and soccer players at the level of the insertion of the Achilles tendon.

The occurrence of these and a hundred related injuries can never be eliminated. The young athlete will always exhibit more enthusiasm than common sense. But they can be limited by good supervision and sensible workout regimens.

Youngsters should always be urged to start gradually so that capabilities meet demands. They must be taught that pain is a warning and that "no pain, no gain" is the motto of the stupid.

They should be taught the basics of good nutrition and the importance of stretching exercises for flexibility. They should be informed of the importance of appropriate footwear and the methods for determining which footwear is appropriate.

Above all they should be encouraged that the purpose of sports is fun, not injury.

What Could I Have Done
to Deserve This?:
The Dancer's Foot

When you think of the dance, what do you think of? A lovely pas de deux, a scintillating leap that defies the laws of gravity (pointy toe)? Well, now think of these from the foot's point of view. For the foot, the dance is a battlefield where the closest you come to victory is a standoff.

If we were to develop a method for destroying the feet, we couldn't do much better than to invent the dance. There is hardly a disaster that can befall the foot that is not S.O.P. for the dancer.

If you are a dancer, you know all this. For every minute you've thrilled an audience, you've spent a half hour attending to your feet and wondering whether the applause is worth the pain.

The agony of foot pain that faces the dancer is summed up in the *en pointe* maneuver. All dancing takes its toll, but there is no doubt that the ballet dancer suffers the worst to fulfill the dream of stardom. We will briefly discuss some other forms of dance before facing the horrors of ballet.

Perhaps the least offensive form of dance, from a foot's point of view, is tap dancing. Emphasizing rhythm and coordination, this form of dance tends to avoid unnatural demands on the foot and therefore most of the serious foot problems.

But even tap extracts a high price in blisters, corns, and callouses. Occasionally a short Achilles tendon will cause an equinus or plantar flexion that will demand treatment. However, these problems are prevented by exercises that stretch the posterior leg muscles and strengthen the anterior muscles.

Modern dance causes more problems than tap, not because its demands are greater but because so much modern dance is done barefoot. A stage is a notorious reservoir of tacks, nails, indescribable but sharp and pointed objects—a regular minefield of career-enders.

Even when the modern dancer avoids these objects, the barefoot approach invites blisters, callouses, fissures, all sorts of additional friction-caused abnormalities, and traumas attending the striking of the floor at the finish of a jeté.

Even those who dance just for fun, the millions of ballroom dancers, pay for their enjoyment. The shoe is almost always the culprit behind problems attacking the ballroom dancer. Both sexes suffer, but it is the woman who wears three- or four-inch heels who most strongly attests to the pain that one who enjoys ballroom dancing is willing to endure. Ankle sprains are not uncommon among young women who dance in such high heels.

When the foot is in so high-heeled a position for such long periods of time under strain so great, the Achilles tendon shortens in rebellion, tightening the posterior leg muscles and threatening the foot with an equinus or plantar-flexed position. This in turn can cause pain in the posterior calf muscles and chronic tendinitis of the Achilles tendon. These problems often respond to a program of stretching exercises.

For millions of Americans the line between dance and exercise has all but evaporated as they have embraced aerobic dancing. While aerobics is undeniably good for your heart, it can be murder on your feet. This applies exponentially to the instructors, who often exercise along with the four or five classes they teach a day.

Typically an aerobic class lasts about an hour. It consists of a warm-up and stretching period, a conditioning period, and a cool-down and stretching period. It is not the nature of aerobics but the length of time for which it is done that is the primary source of the many foot problems it causes. Indeed it has been estimated that 80 percent of the injuries caused by aerobics to the feet and lower legs are the direct result of overuse. The dorsum of the foot is the area most often involved. If those who suffer these traumas had practiced *low-impact* aerobics and had chosen shoes with the care we discuss elsewhere (shoes made for dance areobics, not just any pair of sneakers), they would have avoided the problems that plague them.

Which brings us to classical ballet, the dance equivalent of the Spanish Inquisition. Even before a dancer makes his or her first public appearance, the feet show signs of an assault. Years of dedicated training are required for development of even the basic skills of ballet.

No dancer should begin to dance *en pointe* before having put in a decade of training. Nearly all do. There should be a law against permitting a child to go *en pointe,* but there is no such law. As a result many, perhaps a majority of, ballet dancers suffer from a malady know as knuckling down, in which the toes collapse within the blocked toe of the point shoes. Young dancers, who have not developed sufficient muscle strength and coordination, are particularly vulnerable to this. If a youngster who begins to develop a knuckling condition does not at once refrain from going *en pointe,* there will be no ballet career.

Good technique comes from a slowly learned, proper placement of head, shoulders, hips, knees, and feet. The knowledgeable instructor understands that this takes time and will refrain from pressuring the dancer to "turn out" too early.

There are five basic positions of the feet in ballet. Their common characteristic is the turned-out leg. Here the leg is externally rotated ninety degrees at the hip, resulting in the feet being in a

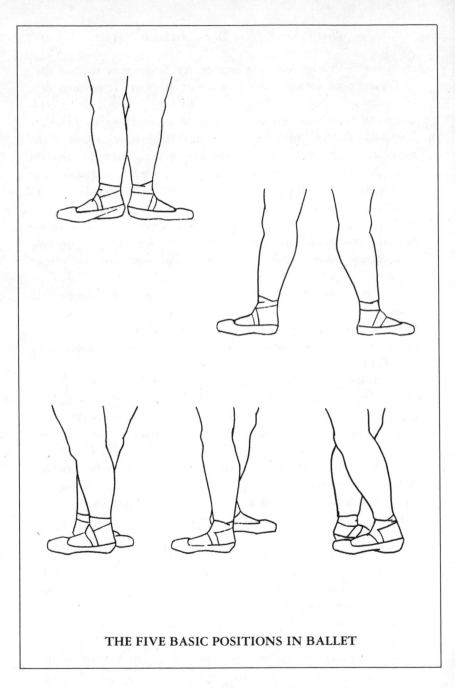

THE FIVE BASIC POSITIONS IN BALLET

straight line, heel-to-heel. All five of the basic positions can be performed with feet flat on the floor, rising high on the balls of the feet, or on the toes.

Young dancers, who usually exhibit more drive than sense, will often attempt to increase turnout, which should occur at the hip, by "screwing the knee." This consists of flexing the knee while moving the feet into the turned-out position and then straightening the knee. This does maximize turnout, but at the expense of rendering likely damage to the medial (inside) of the knee joint. Any child who does this should be told to stop immediately.

A keen adult eye is not sufficient to tell which child will be a great dancer (nothing is), but it can save the child who lacks the physical potential years of wasted training and ultimate heartbreak. General flexibility is mandatory. A flexible person must be pushed to maximum potential to become a dancer; an inflexible person can never become sufficiently flexible no matter what the training.

It is desirable, but not mandatory, that the second and third toes be of equal length. The same can be said of a well-formed arch and stable ankles. Low weight and a lean and lithe body are a starting point; the dancer will be required to become lean and lithe to the point of anorexia.

Knock-knees, severe intoeing gait, internal tibial torsion, gross spinal abnormalities, extremely tight Achilles tendons (which limit dorsiflexion of the foot), and obesity are, at best, warnings that a youngster might better consider another outlet for the creative impulse. All of these are impediments to mastering the basic maneuvers of the dance successfully and each increases the likelihood of failure.

Only the child who cannot live without the dream of a *professional* ballet career should be permitted to follow this path. No child should be pressured into following it. Above all it should be fun, so don't swim upstream.

The classical pointe shoe is both fascinating and considerably more complicated than it looks. It does not come left- and right-footed. Its most notable characteristic is its squared-off toe box.

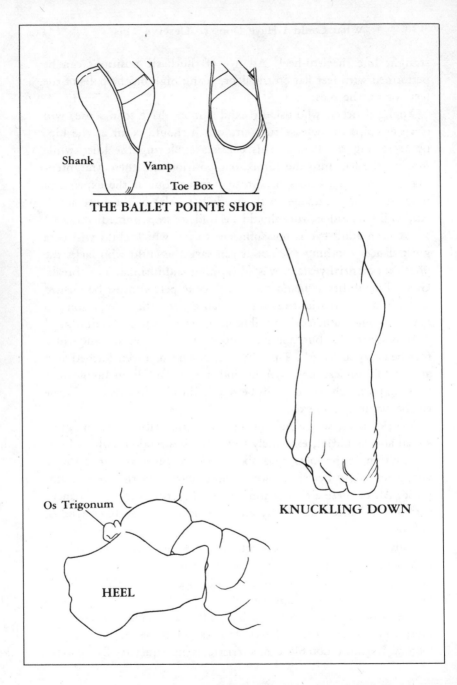

THE BALLET POINTE SHOE

Shank Vamp

Toe Box

KNUCKLING DOWN

Os Trigonum

HEEL

The uppers of the pointe shoes are cut from a special pattern, with the front and back sewn together before the entire upper is stitched. At this point the hard toe box is laminated with layers of fabric and glue. The upper is then placed on a special last and, after tightening, the pleats are formed by hand. After excess material is trimmed, the sole is sewn to the upper and is scored with a sharp cutting tool. This guarantees the traction that the dancer will require. Finally the shoes are oven-dried.

You would think that this would be sufficient. But no dancer has ever been known to be satisfied with a fresh pair of ballet slippers. The finished product of the manufacturer is raw material to the dancer.

Each dancer prepares the slippers in a unique way. First a pink or peach ribbon is sewn inside the slipper, often with dental floss, for strength. The shoes are then softened by hitting them with a hammer, crushing them in slamming doors, and even steaming them over boiling water.

If all goes according to plan, the vamp end of the shoe will end up at the metatarsal-phalangeal joints. The leather, even after softening, is strong and heavy and will ultimately conform to the foot. This is important because the shoe must maintain snug contact with the foot if the dance maneuvers are to be performed safely and successfully. The dancer cannot depend on the orthotic that aids performers in virtually every other arena; it interferes with the sense of the floor that guides the dancer.

With all that can afflict the ballet performer and his or her feet, it is crucial that exercise, preparation, technique, body alignment, and physical condition be perfect. The better the conditioning, the less the chance that the inevitable foot problems will cause permanent damage.

To this end, practice sessions should always include a warm-up activity to increase the heart rate. Brisk walking can accomplish this. Once the heart rate is at a satisfactory level, stretching exercises are performed, with special attention being paid to those muscle groups most used in ballet.

Many of the dancer's foot injuries are traceable to the nature of
the floor surface on which the injuries occur. Very hard surfaces
such as concrete offer no shock absorption and, not surprisingly,
predispose the dancer to shock-related injuries. Tile floors complement the problems of hardness with those of slipperiness. The ideal
surface is made of wood laid over a spongy subsurface of springs or
foam.

Of the specific injuries that plague the dancer, perhaps the *ankle
sprain* is the most common. The usual sprain is of the inversion
type, affecting the ligaments on the lateral (outside) aspect of the
ankle. If the sprain results from only a partial tear of the lateral
ligaments, it will respond well to applications of ice, partial immobilization, and exercises to strengthen the peroneal muscles.
Weight bearing is permitted.

Moderate and severe sprains require more aggressive treatment
and immobilization and can take from four to ten weeks to resolve.
The procedures mentioned above are all required, with additional
strengthening exercises of the muscles being required. Caution
must be exercised, as overstretching an injured area can increase
localized inflammation and damage healing tissues.

(You'll find more information on ankle sprains in the chapter on
foot and ankle injuries.)

Stretching exercises must be slow and steady, lasting for about
ten seconds. *Never* bounce. A most useful exercise for all parts of
the ankle involves placing a towel on the floor perpendicular to the
front of the body. Weight the end of the towel away from the body
with one or two books (but not a heavy weight). Place the heel
firmly on the floor, grasp the towel, and drag it toward the body
by plantar-flexing the toes. Next angle the towel to the left and
place the weights on the far left of the towel. Firmly plant the heel
on the floor and adduct and invert the foot. Then move the foot to
a position of abduction and eversion, pulling the weighted end of
the towel toward the body. This strengthens the peroneal muscle
group on the outside of the leg and ankle. By moving the towel
and weight to the right you can similarly strengthen the medial

aspect of the ankle. Perform this exercise every other day and increase the weight only to the extent that you can do so without pain and not more than once every two weeks. There is no better exercise for strengthening the peroneal muscles.

Tendinitis of the Achilles tendon is an overuse injury characterized by pain and stiffness behind the ankle joint at the posterior aspect of the heel. It responds to heel lifts, three- or four-minute applications of ice, oral anti-inflammatory medication, and ultrasound. Injections of steroids, while occasionally urged by those who do not have the dancer's interest at heart, are contraindicated. In serious cases three or four weeks of rest may be necessary for recovery.

When symptoms abate, an exercise program aimed at strengthening the anterior aspect of the ankle joint and leg may begin. Stretching of the Achilles tendon is best accomplished by standing on a stair with the forefoot and slowly lowering the heel to a level lower than the stair, holding it for fifteen or twenty seconds. Again, never bounce. Toe raises are also helpful in strengthening the tendons. Because the dancer is so attuned to the possibility of dance-caused injury, he or she must never forget that the dancer is not immune to organic problems manifesting themselves in the foot. When Achilles tendinitis is suspected, for example, it is necessary to rule out the possibility of the presence of an accessory ossicle called an *os trigonum.* This fairly common abnormality consists of a small extra bone located at the posterior aspect of the talus. It can mimic, and be confused with, the familiar inflammation of the Achilles tendon. Diagnosis is fairly simple, as the os trigonum can be seen on a lateral X ray of the ankle. In recalcitrant cases surgery may be required.

Stress fractures are precisely what the name implies. A bone is fractured from too much stress on a small area. Dancers are particularly susceptible to stress fractures of the second and third metatarsals and the tibia. Unfortunately such fractures do not always show up on X rays, and it is often necessary to perform a nuclear-imaging bone scan.

It is invariable that a stress fracture requires a cessation of dancing for up to six weeks. It is just as invariable that the dancer will protest this layoff. There is no choice; dancing is stress, and stress is what caused the fracture in the first place. If the dancer refrains from dancing for six weeks, properly supports the foot, and practices low-impact exercises such as cycling, a return to dance within two months is highly likely.

Less serious, and not reasons to take a break from dancing, are *plantar fascitis* and *medial arch pain.* More of a nuisance than a threat, these can usually be controlled by supportive flexible taping, nonsteroidal anti-inflammatory medication, and the usual physiotherapeutic modalities.

Far more of a threat to the ballet dancer is *tendinitis of the flexor hallucis longus tendon.* This tendon must be extremely well developed and healthy if the dancer is to go *en pointe* successfully. Its rupture begins a chain of events that generates a "trigger toe" injury, which causes the first toe to plantar-flex. If the tendon is not ruptured, conservative treatment is usually sufficient for complete recovery. In the case of rupture, surgery is required.

Discussed in other chapters in some detail are the three hallux maladies: *hallux valgus, hallux limitus,* and *hallux rigidus.* The mechanism of deformity is the same for dancers as for nondancers, but the threat is much greater to the former. This is because the affected area, the first metatarsophalangeal, is one of the principal joints called into play in dance. Conservative treatment is always the treatment of choice. Surgery is to be avoided unless absolutely necessary; the results of unsuccessful surgery would be devastating to the dancer.

Two small ossicles under the head of the first metatarsal called sesamoid bones (the medial and lateral) can cause difficulty for the dancer. These bones can fracture after a jeté or can become inflamed from repeated trauma. When inflamed without fracture it is called *sesamoiditis.* It is usually the medial sesamoid bone that is involved. In the case of fracture, termination of dancing, flexible supportive taping, and physiotherapy are helpful. A word of caution: On X rays sesamoid bones can appear to be fractured when in fact they are bipartite sesamoid. It takes a trained eye to differentiate between a true fracture and these abnormally shaped impostors.

Felt padding with an aperture and nonsteroidal anti-inflammatory medication will usually control sesamoiditis. Dancing is permitted. In especially troublesome cases local injection of a steroid can be used.

The array of problems that bother the nondancer, such as skin lesions, hammertoe, fissures, infected ingrown nails, digital problems, and the like can make the dancer's life a living hell. If ever there was a case of "an ounce of prevention," this is it. Careful hygiene, protective devices, taping, and care of the skin are not merely sensible for the dancer but mandatory.

Let us assume that you are, at present, a healthy dancer. There are several things always to keep in mind. In general terms an extremely well-conditioned body and excellent technique can go a long way in preventing many of the physical difficulties that dancers face. Selecting the proper school, knowledgeable instructors, an effective stretching and exercise program, and consideration of stage surfaces are all important to the young dancer.

It is very important to remember that foot surgery is contraindicated for almost all the conditions that can affect the dancer. Only if your career is threatened and there is no alternative should you ever consider surgery. If you do face this situation, get a second and third opinion before the first cut.

Sugar and Spice and
Everything Nice:
The Diabetic Foot

We have referred so often to foot problems associated with diabetes in other chapters that it will come as no surprise that the diabetic faces many, varied, and *very* serious dangers that manifest themselves in the feet. For the diabetic the issue of attention to foot hygiene is not a question of comfort versus annoyance but of life versus death.

We all tend to think of diabetes in terms of its primary effects on blood sugar and related carbohydrate abnormalities, picturing, for example, the diabetic in insulin shock. In reality it is other complications of diabetes—vascular disease, neuropathy, retinopathy, and kidney disease—that far more often kill, maim, and reduce the quality of life of the diabetic. And these are often discovered by the damage they inflict on the foot. Indeed diabetics are hospitalized for foot infections more often than for any other reason.

Diabetes mellitus is a chronic metabolic disease that affects an astonishing one-out-of-twenty Americans. More astonishing is the fact that half of these Americans don't know that they are diabetic. This disease exacts a huge human and financial toll, much of which could be eliminated if more people were tested for it and if those who know they have it were more attentive to their symptoms and their life-style.

Hospitalization for diabetic foot infections alone costs the health-care system (that's all of us) over $200 million a year. The expense for a single amputation is from $8,000 to $12,000 and of course the cost in pain and trauma to the individual is immeasurable.

Diabetes is the leading cause of acquired blindness. The diabetic is two and a half times as likely as the nondiabetic to get heart disease, eight times as likely to contract gangrene requiring amputation, and twenty times as likely to suffer from renal disease. Among people over fifty years old, diabetics are 156 times as likely to develop gangrene as are nondiabetics. Many of these must undergo amputation and 20 percent are dead within two years.

Neuropathy is the constant threatened companion of the diabetic. A third of all diabetics develop distal neuropathy, and 40 percent of diabetic foot lesions are caused by neuropathy. This results from neuropathy's ability to desensitize the diabetic to the pain that warns others to avoid putting pressure on the foot. Since even as low a pressure as five to seven pounds per square inch over a bony prominence can engender ischemic necrosis in less than seven hours, this desensitization has an enormous potential for destruction.

Because the foot manifestations of this disease are so profound and dangerous, it is important that diabetics have as good an understanding of the disease process as possible. Localized foot problems will resist even aggressive treatment if the disease itself is not well controlled. Even though the following paragraphs stray from an explicit discussion of the subject of the foot, the information is presented in an effort to edify the reader.

There are two principal forms of diabetes, and these are distinguished by the age of onset. Juvenile diabetes first appears in children and adolescents, often those of normal or even below-normal

weight. Adult-onset diabetes is nearly always associated with problems of overweight.

In either case diagnosis, treatment, and management come under the venue of the internist, often an internist specializing in the
disease. When the patient follows the internist's instructions, his
prognosis often improves dramatically. It has been estimated that
50 percent of diabetic amputations could be avoided if patients
improved their life-style to lower the risk factors and improved the
surveillance and care of their feet. In one study close supervision,
and the resulting improvement in patient life-style and foot care,
reduced the amputation rate by this amount.

Treatment always consists of increased dietary restriction and
increased exercise and nearly always of the administration of oral
sulfonylurea medications or insulin.

The role of diet in controlling the progression of diabetes proceeds on two fronts. The first is a direct attack on those foods that
worsen the primary diabetic symptoms; the second is a reduction
of foods that contribute to diseases associated with diabetes. For
example every diabetic should cut down his daily intake of satu-
rated fat, which has been indisputably demonstrated to increase the
risk of heart disease that the diabetes itself has already increased. In
general the diabetic is encouraged to replace sugars and fats with
complex carbohydrates. Similarly, high-fiber foods minimize the
increase in blood glucose.

Exercise elevates the level of high-density lipoproteins (HDL),
and this further reduces the risk of heart attack. It also improves
circulation by increasing both cardiac output and peripheral blood
flow. It is mandatory that the diabetic smoker give up his habit
concomitant with his increasing exercise; 90 percent of 35,000 diabetics who require amputation each year are smokers.

Like the improvement in diet and exercise, the medications
available to the diabetic can stabilize and improve their condition,
but they cannot cure their disease.

In noninsulin-dependent diabetics, the sulfonylureas act by di-
minishing insulin resistance in the peripheral tissues and by sen-

sitizing the pancreas to rising blood-glucose levels following meals. In insulin-dependent patients, and in patients resistant to improvement even when diet and exercise schedule are altered, insulin is required.

Medicinal insulin comes in a panoply of types and dosages, and only careful monitoring by internist and patient can ascertain the proper type and dosage.

Here, however, we focus on the effects of diabetes on the foot and the various modalities for addressing these problems.

The mechanism by which vascular disease attacks the diabetic is the same as that discussed in nondiabetic cases. Large and small arteries are involved, but in both cases the disease appears much earlier in the diabetic.

Likewise, arterial insufficiency of the lower extremity, resulting from progressive *atherosclerosis,* energizes a degenerative process that proceeds faster in the diabetic. This occurs chiefly in the aortoiliac vessels, which consist of the distal parts of the aorta, the common iliac artery, and the external iliac artery of the groin area and the femoral, popliteal, and tibial arteries of the leg.

Degenerative symptoms of *large-artery occlusive disease* are intermittent claudication, rest pain, and ulceration. Intermittent claudication is ischemic arterial blood flow resulting from obstruction to the vessel. Secondary to the buildup of lactic acid in the muscle tissue, it manifests itself as a cramping pain that occurs only after walking a short distance. It is relieved by a few minutes' inactivity and gently rubbing the painful calf.

Rest pain, on the other hand, is more serious. Constant lack of blood supply results in continuing discomfort. Manifested as a burning in the foot and increasing with elevation, rest pain usually strikes at night. While it can be relieved by walking, it is, as you might imagine, hell on a good night's sleep.

Small-artery disease results from a thickening of the capillary basement membrane and involves the tiniest vessels. Insulin-dependent diabetics are particularly prone to small-artery disease and are more vulnerable to its effects. Problems that would be of little significance to the nondiabetic, such as callouses, corns, and in-grown toenails, often and easily develop into ulceration, gangrene, and death.

Peripheral neuropathy is another common and extremely dangerous complication of diabetes mellitus. Despite its name, it can affect not only the peripheral nerves but the central nervous system itself.

The principal function of a nerve cell is impulse conduction. Peripheral nerves consist of neurons, Schwann cells, fat, and connective tissue. Many diabetics, perhaps as much as 35 percent, develop a neuropathy that can be demonstrated on clinical examination, with decreased vibratory sense being the most frequent finding. Deep tendon reflexes are diminished or, in some extreme cases, absent.

In addition there can be an accompanying metabolic abnormality of the Schwann cell. The forms of abnormality vary, but common symptoms are impairment of sensation, specifically reaction to heat, cold, pain, and light touch, known as hypoesthesia. Paradoxically some patients suffer an *increase* in sensitivity (hyperesthesia) or abnormal spontaneous sensations occurring without purposeful stimulus. These symptoms can be bilateral or unilateral.

The most common form of diabetic neuropathy is characterized by sensory distal dysfunction. While patients complain of tingling and coldness in the feet, the vital problem, as is so often the case with diabetes, is decreased sensitivity to pain.

While it is only human that the patient fear pain more than its absence, the doctor treating the diabetic is constantly made aware of the survival value of pain. Pain is nature's signal that something is wrong and must be attended to. Without this signal the diabetic often remains unaware of a problem that can kill him. Minor maladies become infected and ulcerated. Pressure of the most minor type turns benign processes into life-threatening ones.

If such problems are left untreated, the small muscles of the foot can atrophy, permitting the powerful long flexor and extensor muscles of the leg to overwhelm the foot. This results in the claw-toe deformity so common among diabetics.

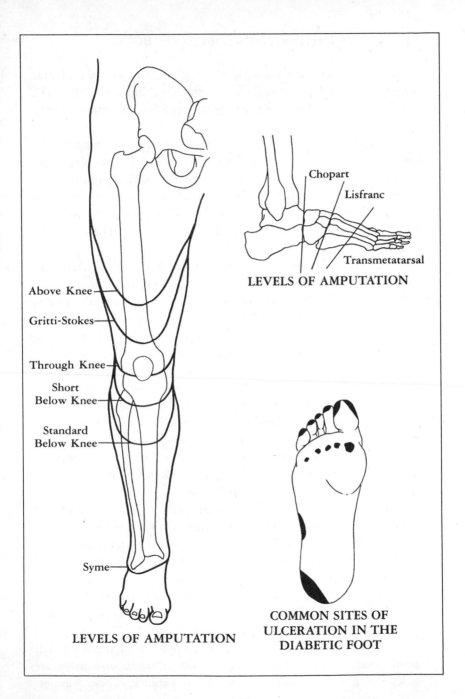

Chopart

Lisfranc

Transmetatarsal

LEVELS OF AMPUTATION

Above Knee

Gritti-Stokes

Through Knee

Short
Below Knee

Standard
Below Knee

Syme

LEVELS OF AMPUTATION

**COMMON SITES OF
ULCERATION IN THE
DIABETIC FOOT**

The ulcer sites often found in the diabetic foot—at the plantar aspect of the heel, the distal ends of the toes, and under all of the metatarsal heads—become as easily infected as they are difficult to treat.

In a minority of cases, physical symptoms are complemented by mental changes that render treatment difficult or impossible. There is, for example, a manifestation of diabetes called eye-foot syndrome, in which neuropathic ulceration and diabetic retinopathy bring with them a sense of euphoria and misunderstanding that convinces the patient that treatment is unnecessary. These patients usually die.

Readers familiar with the history of medicine might recognize the name J. M. Charcot. One of Charcot's lesser known contributions was the identification of a very debilitating osteopathy that is now known as a *Charcot joint.* In his studies of syphilis in the mid-nineteenth century, Charcot noticed that many patients with foot insensitivity, failing to feel the pain that would alert one with a normal foot, will develop one or another of various joint injuries. Since the involved joint never has a chance to heal properly, continued use results in further trauma and degeneration.

People with this problem avail themselves of treatment only when the damage has reached the point where the foot is so swollen that they cannot get into their shoes. Diagnosis is straightforward: The absence of pain and easily identified arterial pulsations immediately identify the problem.

The initial therapy is invariably the removal of all weight and pressure for at least four weeks. The involved limb is kept elevated to control the often profound edema. Elastic bandages and Unna boot applications are invoked in an effort to stabilize the involved joint, and in the most severe cases a plaster cast is used.

Later, accommodative footwear, orthotics, and special insoles are used to support the deformed foot. These are essential if the diabetes and its ravages are to be controlled.

As if all this weren't enough, 30 percent of all diabetics will develop serious dermatological problems. *Diabetic dermopathy* attacks the skin with multiple round red papules. These papules, which for reasons not fully understood occur in men twice as often as in women, are usually asymptomatic and do not require treatment.

Necrobiosis lipoidia diabeticorum, on the other hand, can cause trouble. NLD most often shows up on the shin, though occasionally on the foot. It appears as red papules that enlarge into firm, depressed, waxy-appearing, yellowish-brown plaques. These areas have a reddish-blue raised border and often ulcerate.

This condition is usually bilateral and is both very difficult to treat and most upsetting as a result of its cosmetically unattractive nature. *Bullosis diabeticorum* occurs as a clear blister on the tips of the fingers and toes of middle-aged diabetics.

About 10 percent of all diabetics encounter a yellowing of the palms, soles, and feet. Nearly half develop yellow toenails, usually all ten, with the first two being the most discolored.

While *gangrene* occurs in both dry and wet forms, the former develops more often in the nondiabetic as a result of arterial occlusion. It is the latter that is such a threat to the diabetic, particularly if there is gas present in the infected tissue.

Gas gangrene, caused most often by *Clostridium perfringens,* is an extremely serious threat to life. It often begins with foot infections expressing a redness, warmth, and pussy exudate that does not cause much pain. Plantar abscesses can develop from a tiny crack in the web between the toes, swelling the foot and causing a redness on the sole.

Aggressive antibiotic treatment and foot X rays are mandatory in such cases. Osteomyelitis must be considered carefully and is very difficult to eradicate. On occasion amputation is necessary.

It cannot be stressed too strongly that the most important element in the successful treatment of the diabetic is patient education. The treatment team of internist, nutritionist, and podiatric physician all play a role in educating the diabetic to do the many things that can save his or her life. For all the dangers of diabetes, the well-informed and well-treated diabetic can live a longer, healthier, and more productive life.

Beyond Aspirin:
The Arthritic Foot

Arthritis is so pervasive and so ubiquitously manages to involve the feet that we have already been forced to consider it when discussing problems other than arthritis that have arthritic effects. As the population ages, arthritis will loom even larger, and its crippling and deforming effects will demand even more of our medical efforts and resources.

Arthritis is a chronic, degenerative disease of the cartilage, joints, and bones. Its hallmark is a thickening (hypertrophy) around the joints and a degeneration of the joints. Space between the joints is reduced as the bone becomes thickened and the articular cartilage degenerates. In some cases small spicules of bony osteophytes can be found in the joint space; these are informally known as joint mice, to reflect their ability to inflict further damage of the articular cartilage.

While arthritis can victimize the young, it far more commonly develops with age. It most commonly affects the joints of the foot in the first metatarsal-phalangeal joint and the first metatarsocuneiform joint (at the base of the first metatarsal on the top of the foot).

We have experienced arthritis and known it to be an identifiable entity since before history began, but we know little more about its causes today than we did four thousand years ago.

It does seem to occur most often in the joint subject to wear and tear (that is, the first metatarsal-phalangeals). Arthritis brings with it some degree of destruction and ultimately some degree of loss of function. This in turn causes temporary gait changes that increase the stress placed on other areas of the foot, knee, hip, and lower back. As nearly all who suffer from arthritis discover, the discomfort is worst in the morning, improving with movement and exercise and the passing of waking hours.

Incidentally, the old wives' tale that you can predict the weather by the pain of arthritis is absolutely correct. The changes in humidity that accompany changes in weather affect pressure within the joints; it *does* rain shortly after your knees hurt.

As is often the case with diseases whose causes elude us, we have no cure for arthritis, a reality that is responsible for aspirin being a billion-dollar commodity. There are many prescription non-steroidal medications that lessen inflammation and pain, but it is usually a time-consuming trial-and-error procedure to determine which medication or combination of medications is best for a given person.

Exercise is almost always of benefit, but the exercise must be of a low-impact nature. The last thing damaged joints need is the pounding of the leg against the hard floor.

Proper selection of footwear and well-designed orthotics can help here. Shoes must be customized to the feet they will hold. In some cases, for example, aperture pads can soften pressure on a bony bump on the top of the foot that can otherwise make a comfortable shoe an impossibility. This is a very common symptom of arthritis involving the first metatarsocuneiform joint. As with other abnormalities of the foot, orthotics offer a wonderful defense against collapse of the medial longitudinal arch.

In some cases no footwear can offer hope until surgery reduces anatomical damage caused by the arthritis. In others, even surgery can hope only to eliminate a portion of the effects of the damage and to return only a portion of full functioning.

Not all arthritis is of the sort we have discussed so far. Arthritic joints can be the price for the depositing of crystalline material within the joints. *Gout* is the quintessential example of this.

Realizing that they had given gout a name someone might conceivably remember, the professionals immediately decided that the only acceptable name for the gout's nearest neighbor would, of course, have to be calcium pyrophosphate dihydrate deposition disease (CPDDD). Even the professionals tend to forget this name and refer to the disease as pseudogout.

Gout is the depositing of monosodium urate monohydrate crystals, whereas in CPDDD the crystals are of calcium pyrophosphate dihydrate. Distinguishing between the two is often difficult, and direct examination of the crystals is required for accurate diagnosis.

Symptomatically, gout and pseudogout are pretty much indistinguishable. In both cases the joint is inflamed and will eventually be destroyed if the crystals are permitted to continue accumulating.

True gout presents in two stages: the acute stage and the chronic stage.

An attack of *acute gouty arthritis* is characterized by the sudden onset of dull pain in the first toe joint. The pain quickly becomes excruciating as the toe swells. An attack of this sort is usually self-limiting, tending to abate after two or three really awful days. Do not simply hope it has gone away to bother someone else. If you do nothing at this point, you are virtually certain to suffer again. *Chronic gout,* once a common problem, is less prevalent today; adequate treatment and modern medical and nutritional practices have scored a major victory here. In chronic gout large tophaceous deposits settle in the soft tissues surrounding the joints and ultimately invade and destroy the joints.

Uricosuric drugs, which speed the elimination of uric acid in the urine, are extremely effective for both controlling the situation and preventing further deposits. In extreme cases, when the deposits have destroyed the joints, surgery must be considered.

Osteomyelitis, an infection of the bone caused by a pyogenic organism, is a primary cause of *septic arthritis.* This and numerous other infections can destroy joints. Neuropathy-caused insensitive feet, for example those accompanying Charcot-joint problems in patients with diabetes, often develop such conditions, and diabetics in general, with their decreased ability to fight infection, are prime candidates for septic arthritis.

The list of arthritic-potentiating diseases sometimes seems endless. *Systemic lupus erythematosus,* while primarily a disease of the connective tissue, results in arthritic problems for high numbers of black women in their twenties and thirties. The reason is not known. This has a doubly bad effect because deviations and subluxations unleash the tendency in blacks to develop hyperkeratotic tissue. Tender, slowly healing ulcers of the leg often develop near the medial and lateral malleolus around the ankle joint.

The patient typically complains of joint pains without any external signs of localized inflammation, redness, or heat. Indeed, in the early stages, even X rays fail to identify the problem. Fortunately the deformity of the joints caused by systemic lupus erythematosus is easily reduced or rectified.

Unfortunately such is not the case with *rheumatoid arthritis.* The joint is subluxated but not destroyed. Nonetheless, forcible straightening of the joint will typically fail to prevent a return to the deformed position. Because there is no bone or cartilage destruction, the problem is more one of nonerosive arthropathy than one of true arthritis.

Patients with rheumatoid arthritis have within their blood serum a substance called rheumatoid factor (RF). There are a group of diseases called seronegative spondyloartopathies that also have associated arthritic-joint changes but that do not exhibit RF (thus the "seronegative"). Examples of these are ankylosing spondylitis, psoriatic arthritis, and Reiter's syndrome.

In *ankylosing spondylitis* foot involvement is minimal. But *psoriatic arthritis* often presents symmetrical involvement of the small joints of the toes. There is an erosion of bone, especially from the distal phalanx, and the toes take on a sausagelike appearance. Diagnosis is often delayed by a confusion of the disease with a similar-appearing fungus infection. Once a diagnosis is made, treatment is conservative.

Reiter's syndrome is a triad of overlapping symptoms: conjunctivitis, urethritis, and asymmetrical arthritis. It affects the foot primarily in the heel, though sausage toes and painful retrocalcaneal bursa are frequent corollaries. The heel is attacked at both the plantar and the posterior aspects, with erosion causing the appearance of a poorly defined heel spur.

Rheumatoid arthritis, in general, can be said to be a systemic disease of unknown origin that often involves the foot, causing a disabling joint destruction and deformity. It is estimated to victimize over five million Americans. In most cases there is bilateral and symmetrical involvement of the foot, particularly the forefoot. The first joint to be affected is often the fifth of the lateral metatarsophalangeal joints. As the disease involves the remaining metatarsophalangeal joints, the foot becomes swollen and ultimately deformed.

Swelling at the level of the proximal phalangeal joints of the toes is a common symptom and sign of rheumatoid arthritis. Often this is accompanied by a severe hallux valgus deformity that forces the first toe to drift laterally either under or over the lesser toes.

Because of the laxity of the tendons, the forefoot tends to splay under the pressure of body weight. This initiates a chain reaction in which the development of claw toes with the typical swan-neck deformation is joined by a clawing of the lesser toes. This leads the plantar fat pad to shift distally, exposing the plantar aspect of the metatarsals to pressure and irritation. Large, painful callouses develop under the metatarsal heads, and rheumatoid nodules can assault the foot tendons, causing pain and disability.

While rheumatoid arthritis usually spares the ankle joint, it often affects the midfoot and rearfoot and reduces joint space in these areas.

Because the loss of the medial longitudinal arch is associated with subtalar joint involvement, people with rearfoot deformity often respond very well to orthotics. Likewise, people with forefoot deformity can he helped by metatarsal pads. Crepe and rubber-soled shoes are advised for their impact-reducing qualities and their ability to limit trauma to the foot. Similarly, the use of crutches reduces pressure. If claw toes present a problem, extra-depth shoes that accommodate the toes are helpful.

Selecting a proper athletic shoe is very important for the active arthritic patient. It can sometimes be difficult to find a shoe of adequate width to accommodate the deformed feet. The fifth meta-tarsal area (on the outside of the foot) should never land over the side of the shoe.

A shoe with Velcro-type closures will help ease the pain of tying laces in patients with arthritis of the hands. A flaring of the outsole both at the heel and toe area will increase overall stability. A firm heel counter will prevent unnecessary medial and lateral motion. Sole flexibility will aid in the painful push-off stage of gait. An air-cushioning system built into the shoe will attenuate shock. Most of the better shoes have support for the arch that will help prevent pronation.

Interestingly these features are not normally found in walking or aerobic-type shoes, but are found in running shoes.

It is crucial that one suffering rheumatoid arthritis persevere with gentle exercises, both active and passive. These are necessary if the full range of motion is to be maintained.

Unfortunately physiotherapeutic modalities have proven of limited value. Treatment of the disease consists primarily of ongoing attempts to limit or eradicate pain, to correct and prevent deformity, and to preserve and restore function.

Systemic treatment of the disease is in the hands of the rheumatologist, whose first line of defense is the use of salicylates. Nonsteroidal anti-inflammatories offer help in some cases, while gold and other agents are occasionally successful in arresting the disease before joint destruction occurs. Injections of steroids can reduce pain, but restraint must be exercised in their use.

There is an extensive array of surgical procedures available for correction of deformities caused by rheumatoid arthritis. Most common is correction of severe hallux valgus deformity. In some cases all of the metatarsal heads must be resected in order to resolve extremely painful and diffuse plantar callosities. Implants must be used with caution in patients with rheumatoid arthritis. If there is significant rearfoot involvement, it is often necessary to surgically fuse the joints.

The onset of *juvenile rheumatoid arthritis* can come at any time up to the mid-teen years. It is three times as common in girls as in boys. It makes its appearance in one of three major modes of onset: systemic, polyarticular, and pauciarticular. The first of these is found in equal numbers of boys and girls and makes its presence known through fever, anthralgia without swelling, and, in about 90 percent of the cases, rash. The rash is usually on the torso, but can occur on the face, neck, palms, or soles. It is flat or only slightly raised and does not itch.

Systemic-onset juvenile rheumatoid arthritis can bring myocarditis with it, and this, as a result of its ability to engender heart failure, can threaten life.

The sign that is important with the polyarticular-onset of the disease is the painful swelling of four or more joints, most often the joints of the knees, wrists, ankles, or elbows. The fever is usually low-grade but chronic.

Pauciarticular onset marks the beginning of nearly half of the cases and lacks significant fever or heart involvement. In girls the site is often the knee. The greatest, though uncommon, threat is blindness due to iridocyclitis.

Medical management of juvenile rheumatoid arthritis entails recognition, prompt treatment of any eye or heart involvement, and prevention of deformity from the progressive polyarthritis. Medications such as salicylates, nonsteroidal anti-inflammatories, and steroids are indicated in many specific instances.

Rest and exercise must be carefully balanced if efforts to reduce pain and inflammation and to improve joint function are to be successful. High-impact sports must be avoided, but activities such as swimming are excellent. These increase flexibility and strength, both in the muscles and in the ligaments that surround the joints, and increase bone strength. Immobility and disuse are the great danger of arthritis (once the disease itself is treated), and exercise is the antidote for these.

In many cases it is best to have the exercise program developed by a professional who becomes familiar with the specific patient. This is necessary because exercise for the arthritic must walk the line between inactivity and activity that will damage fragile parts. One example: joint cartilage, which is often damaged by arthritis, requires nourishment by synovial fluid. This nourishment is facilitated by movement, but inappropriate movement can be destructive. A specialist trained in the exercise needs of the arthritic can customize a program that attains the good and avoids the bad.

Undoing joint damage is, in fact, the primary task of exercise. Stretching exercises are designed to increase a joint's range of motion and lengthen tendons. Range-of-motion exercises can be accomplished by patients themselves (active) or by another person helping the patient perform the movements (passive). Range-of-motion exercises incrementally improve the ability of the joints to do their job and strengthen the muscles that move the joints. Isometric exercises, in which you push against an immovable object, offer a way of strengthening the muscle without putting too much stress on the joint. Endurance activities, such as walking and bicycling, serve as an interest-maintaining adjunct to swimming and support cardiovascular fitness.

The psychological and social benefits of exercise are, for one with arthritis, almost as great as the physical benefits. Arthritis can impose restrictions on mobility and life-style that threaten to severely limit options and lower self-esteem. Exercise makes possible the achievement of goals and, when done with others, social interaction that counteracts these threats.

Save for the situations in which the joints are inflamed or hot, one who suffers from arthritis or, particularly, rheumatoid arthritis should exercise twice a day for the rest of his or her life. For this reason variety is, as we have suggested, crucial.

Because it is so important, it is necessary to find the best times of the day for your exercise. If you fit your program into your lifestyle, you will find that it is more easily integrated into your daily life. Often it is best to choose times that complement the times when medication is taken.

A warm-up period is essential for all who exercise, but it is crucial for the arthritic. This should be followed by a period of slow, controlled movement that prepares the body for more demanding exercise. A hot bath or shower followed by a massage is both healthy and an incentive.

Above all it is necessary to learn proper form. Exercise done improperly is worse than no exercise at all. Begin at whatever level is comfortable for you and don't worry about those who can do more. Soon so will you. It is important not to overdo any exercise program. If postexercise pain lasts longer than a couple of hours, you may very well be exercising excessively. Use a slow, steady rhythm and breathe deeply and rhythmically. Wear warm clothing and avoid becoming chilled during your session.

We will not pretend that all exercise is fun. The result, not the process, is usually what makes exercise worthwhile. Music or books on tape can reduce boredom and enable you to accomplish two things at once.

Do not be discouraged. Progress might be slow at first, but with perseverance results can be spectacular.

Your Feet Get Old Faster
Than the Rest of You:
The Geriatric Foot

The American population is getting older; fewer babies are being born than were a decade or two ago, therefore the population's average age is increasing.

The portion of the population that is increasing most rapidly is the one over sixty-five. This group gets bigger not merely as a result of decrease in birthrate but also as a result of medical advances that prolong longevity.

And the part that gets oldest first is the feet. Many of the diseases we discuss attack the old disproportionately, and many of the surgical cures are risky when performed on the elderly. Thus the foot problems of the elderly have become sufficiently great to be a subject, and a specialty, of their own.

Even the older person who has been fortunate enough to avoid serious illness will have feet that show the assault of six or seven decades of being pounded into the ground. Between 75 and 95 percent of the elderly have foot problems of one sort or another. They suffer the entire catalog of foot problems: corns, callouses, bunions, ingrown nails, heel difficulties, arch pain, all sorts of localized arthritic changes, trophic skin changes, sensory nerve dysfunction, ulcers—the list could go on and on.

People who are institutionalized often have less painful problems than the more active older man or woman, but they still require supervision and care. The lessened activity reduces stress on the feet, but other problems, such as nail disorders, can present difficulties. Good foot care is perhaps more important for the elderly than for any other group. The sense of independence of the old person is under constant assault, and painful feet offer no foundation for a sense of independence. This leads many older people to attempt self-medication that is neither advisable nor likely to solve the problems they are meant to solve. Poor vision, joints stiff from arthritis, and obesity, all problems found disproportionately among the old, make self-care virtually impossible even when people know what they are doing (which they often don't).

Moreover the effects of poor self-care can be far worse than a mere failure to correct the problem they were meant to correct. Many diseases of the elderly reduce circulatory efficiency and leave one vulnerable to infections that would cause no problem in a healthy person. The improperly cut corn, callous, or nail can engender such an infection. Even simple dry skin, a common condition among the elderly, can cause fissures that, if improperly treated, can invite bacterial invasion and cause infection.

So, as you can see, a simple problem can have results as catastrophic as amputation. Fortunately when treated by the podiatrist, such problems have simple cures. The application of a good skin lotion, for example, will keep the skin smooth and fissure-free by preventing loss of moisture.

Likewise, soaking the feet before applying the lotion will not only enhance the lotion's effects but will feel pleasant and be relaxing. Just make sure the water isn't too hot. An added benefit is that it allows the elderly to do something to help themselves.

The aging process entails a loss of plantar fat tissue that can predispose one to the painful heel syndrome. Loss of fat under the metatarsal heads can lead to very painful plantar callosities.

Even the gait changes as we age. This is seen most clearly in the "old man's walk." As we reach old age, our stride shortens, cadence decreases, and swing-to-stance ratio lessens. These changes all tend to decrease the force load carried by the foot. Actually this is all to the good if a person accepts that he can do less than he once could. But many people are not wise and continue to make demands that the foot can no longer meet.

Pain in the forefoot is usually due to corns on the toes, callouses on the bottoms of the feet, toenail disorders, bunions, or locked joints. Because the elderly are often not sufficiently good surgical candidates to justify surgery for problems that do not threaten life, palliative measures must be used.

There is an array of products for these problems, ranging from the marvelous to the dangerous. Aperture pads, moleskin and its modern equivalents, lamb's wool, foam-rubber inserts, and crest pads for under the toes are all available at many drugstores.

Pads with acid or liquid caustic agents should not be used without professional supervision. The consequences of chemical burns for a person with decreased circulation can be devastating. Lamb's wool, on the other hand, is entirely safe and very effective. It compresses better than cotton, is absorbent, and molds easily to any size and shape. It is very effective in easing the pain of corns between the toes and a wonderful buffer, when placed under the plantar aspect, preventing the buildup of painful callouses. Crest pads placed under the toes and looped over the top can relieve the pressure of corns on the ends of the toes.

The elderly are plagued by nail problems that come in the form of thickened, brittle, and discolored nail plates. *Onychomycosis,* a fungus infection of the nail plate, can be the cause of all of these symptoms. The elderly often have physical problems making nail care difficult, and they should not attempt to care for their own nails. A podiatrist will carefully cut the nails, remove any dead, thickened skin, and reduce the nail plates by grinding them with a drill. Even when these nail problems cause no pain, they should be attended to. They are unsightly and also increase the likelihood of infection.

Problems and discomfort associated with bunion (*hallux valgus*) and locked joint (*hallux rigidus*) are often helped as much by improving the shoes as by direct medical intervention. You can accommodate a painful bunion by increasing the width of a shoe (a process any shoemaker can perform) or buying wider shoes. A shoe with a stiff and thickened sole can alleviate the pain of hallux rigidus, and shoes with extra depth and an accommodative insert can relieve pressure by substituting for lost plantar-fat-pad material.

It is most common to find older patients with a bump on the top of the foot at the level of the first metatarsocuneiform joint. This is caused by *osteoarthritis* and can make fitting a shoe difficult. The answer here is one or more felt pads placed under the tongue of the shoe. These pads absorb the pressure that would otherwise focus on the bump.

The *heel pain* we mentioned comes in many forms and has many causes: heel spurs, lack of heel fat pad, bursa at the posterior aspect of the heel, plantar fasciitis, and Achilles tendon bursitis are some of the more common. Many of these heel problems can be alleviated by simple cushioning and slightly elevating the heel. Any diminution of fat pads can be helped by augmentation with foam-rubber inserts. Plastic heel cups, both rigid and flexible, can greatly reduce the pain of Achilles tendon bursitis and tender heels. A SACH heel (Solid Ankle Cushioning Heel), a compressible heel made of soft materials such as crepe or sponge rubber, and sometimes a top lift of hard rubber, is very effective in resistant cases.

People with thickened medial and lateral plantar heel callouses also respond well to heel cups of various types.

In all cases it is crucial to remember that when a foot problem is caused by a disease such as diabetes, rheumatoid arthritis, or gout, it is not enough to treat the symptom, even if it is the only symptom.

Trauma almost invariably presents a greater threat to the elderly than it does to the young. Older patients often suffer from excessive swelling even before a trauma, and the swelling resulting from a trauma can last for months. The elastic bandages that are so helpful for the younger patient are difficult for the old to apply. Elastic stockings are usually preferable.

We have mentioned a few specific conditions for which proper selection of shoes can alleviate foot problems in the elderly. There are many other situations in which proper selection of footwear does not merely alleviate a problem but precludes its developing in the first place. As a rule, the geriatric patient is less concerned with appearance than is the younger patient. Pain has a way of overcoming vanity.

The first thing that an older person should look for in a shoe is good support to relieve arch strain. Next comes flexible uppers to relieve pressure on the toes. The insole should be soft enough to cushion the plantar structures and provide a soft buffer between foot and ground.

Fit is crucial, and difficult. Many older people have foot deformities that shoe manufacturers have not anticipated. Sometimes a tradeoff must be accepted. Bunions and hammertoes, for example, require a wider shoe than the individual would otherwise wear, even if this means some looseness at the heel. The secondary problem can be dealt with separately (for example, butterfly foam-rubber heel pads can provide heel grasp and overcome the wideness introduced by the solution to the hammertoes).

Many older patients prefer open-heeled shoes with adjustable straps. This is fine for summer, but raises obvious problems in the winter.

In some instances shoes with extra width, extra depth, open heels, and the like, will not get the job done. In such cases custom shoes may be the only alternative.

Custom shoes are made from an impression of your foot. This impression is filled with plaster of Paris, which in turn becomes a mold that is the last over which the shoe is made. Because the shoe is made to a mold of your unique foot, it can accommodate any deformity or abnormality your foot may exhibit.

We won't pretend these shoes will win fashion award after fashion award. Often referred to as space shoes, they trade beauty for comfort. They can be very comfortable and allow a person to continue walking and enjoy mobility who would otherwise be at least partially disabled. Now the bad news: They are expensive.

If there is anyone who can benefit from a visit to the podiatrist, it is the geriatric patient. Indeed everyone over sixty-five should consider routine visits essential. Foot care should be included in all health-insurance policies. Often such policies, whether governmental or private, strictly limit foot coverage. This is shortsighted. There are few more cost-effective measures than prevention of a problem that will be frightfully expensive to solve if it is not prevented.

But, most importantly, good treatment of the elderly is only required by fairness. And common sense. We will all get old. Or at least the lucky among us will.

Strange Bedfellows—the Laser, Arthroscopic Surgery, and Your Feet: Newer Modalities

In the early part of this century a report that was to change medical education from top to bottom concluded that if you were sick or injured, you were best off staying as far away from a doctor as you could. While preceding centuries had provided a few geniuses whose discoveries made modern medicine possible, the doctor-in-the-street was as likely to kill you as save you.

You probably know that the red-and-white stripes of the barber pole represent the blood and bandages of the unfortunate patient, but you may not know about a thousand "cures" so horrible that you should consider yourself lucky to be ignorant of them.

Fortunately things have changed. After the reformation of the medical school and the introduction of the scientific method, a doctor's "knowledge," formerly a hodgepodge of superstition and nonsense, became real knowledge, a more or less accurate view of the way things work.

This is not to say there were not, or are not, large areas of ignorance, or that the doctor can cure anything that should happen to ail you. But for the past fifty years scientific knowledge of the body has grown continuously, and your body is the beneficiary of this knowledge.

Particularly that area of your body that interests us: your feet. In the last fifteen years alone, the armamentarium of weapons available to the clinician has been enlarged enormously. Technological advances in far-flung fields have given us a myriad of ways of curing foot problems before which we had formerly been powerless. Here we shall examine some of the most important of these advances.

Lasers

While lasers do not provide the panacea for all foot problems they are sometimes represented as providing in advertisements, they do offer remarkable relief for those for which they are appropriate.

The term *laser* is an acronym for *l*ight *a*mplification by *s*imulated *e*mission of *r*adiation. What that means is this: An excited atom is struck by a photon (a "particle" of light; more precisely the basic unit of light energy). In response the atom emits a photon and then relaxes into its normal, unexcited state. The photon emitted in this collision mirrors the wavelength and direction of the original photon and strikes another atom, thereby replicating the original collision. A sort of chain reaction begins, and we harness this energy and directionality in order to deliver it to precisely the spot on the body in need of alteration.

Specific types of lasers are named for the essential element or compound used to produce the atomic action. Carbon dioxide, argon, and ruby are examples. Whatever the substance, the method is more or less the same.

Mirrors are placed at each end of a chamber. A small portion of photons is redirected through the active medium (the substance) and this stimulates further emissions, creating the laser light.

The mirrors are not identical. While one is a totally reflecting mirror, the other offers only partial reflection, allowing a certain amount of light to be transmitted through while reflecting the rest to the totally reflecting mirror at the other end of the chamber. The escaping laser light is directed through an articulated arm and into a surgical handpiece. Finally an optical lens focuses the beam to an astonishing amount of precision.

The theory of simulated emission that makes all this possible was first proposed by Albert Einstein (who else?) over seventy years ago. However it was not until recently that theory could be translated into practical application.

The choice of type of laser is not determined merely by color preference. Each type has a different effect on tissue, permitting the doctor to use the laser most closely approximating the needs of a specific patient and problem.

The carbon dioxide laser, the most commonly used in podiatric situations, has a wavelength that is heavily absorbed by water. When so absorbed, the wavelength produces a vibration that causes water to boil and vaporize. Since the soft tissues of the body can contain up to 90 percent water, the specificity of the carbon dioxide laser makes it an invaluable tool of the podiatrist.

The light emitted by the carbon dioxide laser is monochromatic and invisible to the naked eye (though the addition of a helium neon laser produces a pure-red directional beam). It can be focused and concentrated into an incredibly small area because, unlike the forms of light familiar to us, it does not diffuse significantly with distance. Where a regular light bulb produces light of many different wavelengths and spreads out over a room, a laser can come within inches of hitting a target on the moon. As a result, where a bulb of 20 watts is barely capable of providing reading light, a laser of 20 watts is surgically powerful.

Argon lasers are used in eye surgery to coagulate retinal bleeding and to repair retinal detachments. Neodymium-YAG lasers, which produce a beam visible to the naked eye, are used to coagulate large and deep gastrointestinal bleeders and to treat deep tumors. The reader will be glad to know that we need not consider these here.

The carbon dioxide laser, often used in podiatric surgery, comes closest to matching the general public's idea of what a surgical laser is. Used primarily for vaporization of soft tissues, it makes an exceedingly fine and narrow incision, how fine and narrow depending on the power density of the laser and its contact time.

Because the laser can make an incision and coagulate vessels of 0.5 millimeters in diameter, it is often referred to as a bloodless scalpel, a term that is accurate for all intents and purposes, if not literally true.

It is not always the case that the podiatrist wishes to avail himself of the laser's focusing ability. When a vessel is larger in diameter than 0.5 millimeters, the blood it carries will not coagulate and will bleed into the wound. In such cases the water content of the blood threatens to bleed into the wound as well and to undo the work for which the laser is used. In such cases the laser beam is defocused, thereby coagulating a larger area at a small expense in intensity.

Laser surgery is a powerful weapon in the battle against a host of other foot abnormalities. Skin lesions, fungal nail lesions, ingrown nails, and even unwanted tattoos fall before the power of the beam. Bone abnormalities, however, are not amenable to laser rectification, because bone has a high mineral and low water content.

In general the advantages of laser surgery result from the basic characteristics of the laser and its interaction with tissue. Since the laser leaves the area being operated on bloodless, the view of the problem is unimpeded. The laser vaporizes not merely the affected tissue but also bacteria, fungi, and viruses that could cause problems worse than the one being solved. The wound is, in other words, automatically sterilized.

Medically less important, but of equal importance to the patient, is the fact that laser surgery produces less pain and fewer scars than do traditional modes of surgery. It is less traumatic in terms of pain and scarring as a result of its astonishing specificity;

adjacent tissue is not damaged and therefore does not cause pain or scarring.

However, these same virtues can lead people to demand laser surgery when it is not indicated. More than one such patient has stormed out of a podiatric office, convinced that the podiatrist simply didn't know his lasers. In fact, while lasers are a wonderful adjunct to regular surgical techniques, it must always be remembered that they have their limits.

Moreover laser surgery is not without its risks, even when such surgery is indicated. The most common danger is burn; the very power that makes the laser so potent can cause trouble when things go wrong. In truth it is not the laser itself that causes the mishaps—like all tools and weapons, it is, in itself, passive—but the various operating-room personnel. A wrong move by anyone, from the patient to the attending assistants to the surgeon, can cause a burn in whatever tissue becomes the target of the laser. It is not unknown for a misdirected beam to set a surgical drape on fire. (For this reason all surgical drapes are moistened.) Beams reflected off concavities can be misdirected and burn whatever they happen to strike. Faulty equipment has resulted in electrocution, and reflection of the laser off polished instruments has been the source of burns. (Thus, ebonized or brushed-finish instruments are used.)

Want more? You may know that the world is a tough place, but bet you weren't even counting the danger of inhaling a laser plume, the superheated water vapor and particulate cellular matter created upon impact of laser and tissue. The pulmonary system is not fond of this "smoke."

The reader may come out from under the bed now. Fortunately most of these dreadful mishaps are a thing of the past. Experience has forced constant improvement of laser operating techniques, and accidents are now rather rare. Personnel use protective eyewear specific to the frequencies of the laser (as does the patient), and equipment is checked constantly. Finally operating-room vacuum systems have been beefed up to counteract the dangers of laser plume.

Arthroscopy

Prior to the mid-seventies, arthroscopic surgery—surgery performed inside a joint, using miniature instruments through a very small incision—while not unknown, was quite uncommon. The size of the active elements of the equipment was to the parts being operated on as a flagpole is to a straw, and the resulting failure rate reflected this fact. Now, however, refinements have made this a whole new game, and the arthroscope is frequently used for diagnosis, permitting repairs of joint problems once thought incurable.

Particularly for diagnosis, the instrument permits the surgeon to see where he formerly could only guess. The arthroscope carries light to the actual site of the problem and transmits a picture of the abnormality to the surgeon. Arthroscopy, the technical name for this procedure, has been the beneficiary of ever-accelerating improvements in lens development and the development-transmitting tubes of a wide range of sizes. This has enormously improved our ability to home in on a problem area and to view it from a host of angles.

Arthroscopy is now routinely used for knee- and ankle-joint repairs. While the best-known beneficiaries of arthroscopic advances have been highly paid athletes whose careers have been extended, in some cases by many years, for every such athlete there are a thousand average people whose lives have been improved by the arthroscopic eradication of knee and ankle problems. At present arthroscopic diagnosis is not used in the smaller joints of the foot, but this will no doubt cease to be true in the near future.

Arthroscopy of the ankle is indicated for various loose and detached bodies, long-standing posttraumatic pain, injuries to the ligaments, chondral fractures, and osteochondral fractures.

Diagnosis of these entails threading the light cable to the site. Once this is accomplished, the surgeon gets a view of the affected area far sharper than that of an ordinary television program. The image can be transmitted to an eyepiece or to a monitor made specially for this purpose.

Not surprisingly the key element in the arthroscopic device is the bulb. Most commonly used is the tungsten lamp, which generates a color temperature of 2,900 K degrees while operating on only 150 watts. Metal halide bulbs are more expensive but double the temperature attained and provide a much whiter light. As with most other things, top dollar brings the best results; xenon lamps, the most expensive, operate at the same 300 watts as do the halide bulbs, but provide 6,000 K degrees and the brightness of daylight. The two most commonly used camera systems using these bulbs are the saticontube and the CCD chip camera.

The actual practice of arthroscopy is as much art as science, and as is the case with other arts, the results are determined to a great extent by the practitioner's technical skill. Arthroscopy of the ankle, which is virtually always performed in the operating room, is always preceded by administration of an anesthesia: local, regional, or general, as the situation demands. As in any joint surgery, sterile precautions and operating drapes are mandatory. Once all is in place, the sequence of events will be determined by the practices of the particular surgeon.

After taking note of the topographical anatomy and marking important landmarks on the skin, some surgeons will use a mid-thigh pneumatic tourniquet. With the patient in a supine position, the ankle capsule is distended by infiltration of a normal saline solution.

At this point a small stab incision is made through the skin to allow arthroscopic entry. A sharp cannulated trocar is used to pierce the soft tissue. Holding the cannula in place, the surgeon removes the sharp trocar and replaces it with a dull obturator that is used to penetrate the deeper synovium and enter the joint space.

The surgeon knows that he is working inside the joint when he sees the saline solution begin to flow out. When this occurs, he removes the obturator and inserts the arthroscope through the cannula and into the joint. At this point the light cable and the camera are connected to the arthroscope and the image of the problem area can be seen on the monitor.

Throughout the ensuing procedure the joint is kept distended with a constantly flowing saline solution, the source of which are bags of the solution on the intravenous pole above the patient. Gravity forces the solution through an ingress tube, and this and another cannula guarantee that the joint is irrigated throughout the procedure.

Here the serious cutting begins. The surgeon brings into play an armamentarium of tools he has mastered throughout his career. After carefully and systematically examining the joint in order to decide the appropriateness of various tools, he will choose among such hand-powered instruments as scissors, probes, knives, forceps, rasps, and files and a wide selection of battery or electrically operated devices.

While such an impressive, not to say terrifying, array of instruments for cutting tissue and bone may seem intimidating, the very range and variation of these instruments permits a delicacy that translates into surgical success.

For example, cutters are used for excision of synovial and fibrous tissue, while burrs are used for abrasion therapies. These and all of the other instruments represent the state-of-the-art of the medical-tool trade, and the patient is the beneficiary of the great advances permitted by recent improvements in metallurgy and fine honing.

When the arthroscope is removed and the procedure is completed, the ankle is manually compressed to force out whatever fluid remains. A simple suture is usually sufficient to close the portal of entry and, once a soft compression dressing is applied, the patient is ready to bear weight.

In some cases the postoperative situation is more complex. After a transchondral fracture is treated or an abrasion arthroplasty is performed, for example, it is necessary to place the patient on a continuous passive-motion machine for about six days. Furthermore the wound must not be required to bear weight for six weeks or more. Compensating for this annoyance is the fact that there is often a dramatic relief from pain, as well as an impressive improvement in the range of motion, immediately following the operation.

This is particularly common with posttraumatic arthritis and adhesive capsulitis.

Magnetic Resonance Imaging (MRI)

Now in wide use, MRI is perhaps the most important advance in evaluation of a variety of musculoskeletal processes and disorders in the past fifty years. It is superior to X rays and other evaluative modalities in its ability to display inherent contrast distinctions between tissues. Moreover MRI, unlike the X ray, for example, permits manipulation of image during examination. In other words the area of expected pathology can be highlighted for a much sharper view of the problem area than is the case with previous methods.

Fortunately Magnetic Resonance Imaging works perfectly well on one whose idea of electrical engineering is turning on a radio. For the more technically inclined, it is worth pointing out that MRI uses low-energy radio waves to produce its images. Production of the image requires four components: (a) magnetic nuclei; (b) a strong static magnetic field; (c) coils for transmission and reception of radio frequency waves; and (d) magnetic gradients (small magnetic fields with known, carefully controlled spatial variation). The actual image is reconstructed from observed frequency wave signals by use of a computer in a manner similar to that used in computerized tomography (CT) scans.

The patient is placed in a homogeneous, high-strength magnetic field. This causes the hydrogen nuclei to align with the field in much the same manner that a compass needle aligns with the earth's magnetic field. The resulting magnetic field is about 0.1 telsa. The relative strength of the field becomes apparent when we consider that the strength of the earth's magnetic field at the surface of the United States is 1/20,000th of this. This signal is maintained for as long as the radio frequency wave pulse is "turned on," causing absorption of energy by nuclei and a resulting change in their alignment.

Once the radio frequency wave pulse is removed, the nuclei return to their original alignment in the external magnetic field at virtually the speed of light. In doing so they radiate energy, and it is this measurable emitted energy that can be detected by a receiver. Two constants, termed T1 and T2, which are different for each type of body tissue, indicate the rate at which the absorbed energy is lost and the hydrogen nuclei realign themselves with the cessation of the radio stimulation. Other properties, such as the hydrogen-nuclei density of the tissue and the vectors of nuclear motion, contribute to an enhanced image. The strength of the signal, incidentally, is proportional to the nuclear density, the nuclear motion, and the relaxation times of T1 and T2.

Because a single pulse sequence can fail to distinguish between normal and abnormal tissue, more than one sequence is always used. Increasingly accurate images, and decreasing probability of error, is obtained as additional sequences are checked. Variation of the magnetic field applied to the tissue identifies location with increasing accuracy, and selective excitation—the excitation of only an exceedingly thin cross-section of tissue—makes possible axial discrimination of the tissue. This process is repeated many times, and the resulting different projections permit accurate reconstruction.

Magnetic Resonance Imaging is among the sagest of diagnostic tests, but it is not totally without risk. Care must be taken to prevent magnetic objects, such as watches, jewelry, and scissors, from being taken into the scanning room. Interestingly the sorts of metal objects used in foot surgery, such as wires, staples, screws, and plates, are usually nonmagnetic and therefore safe. People with pacemakers are not candidates for MRI.

Patient intolerance can be another source of problems. MRI can often take over an hour, and the restrictive nature of the scanning space containing the patient can cause discomfort.

However, for people willing to endure the discomfort, the diagnostic rewards are very great. The tissue contrast in an MRI is dramatically clear. Fat, muscle, nerve, cartilage, ligaments, blood vessels, and bone are virtually as distinguishable from each other as they are when observed directly. As a result MRI has great clinical value in evaluating bone marrow disorders, bone tumors, osteomyelitis, and infection and massing in the soft tissue.

Because of its high cost, MRI is rarely used in diagnosis of fractures or in routine screenings. But when less expensive modalities are not up to the job, MRI is a medical godsend.

Part Two

Common Foot Problems
Involving the Skin

What is waterproof, comes in different colors, varies in thickness, stretches easily, and protects us from the elements? A plastic raincoat? Wrong. The integument, the skin. It is the first anatomical structure encountered on the journey into the human foot. The outer layer, the epidermis, has no blood supply of its own and gets its nutrition from the deeper layer, the dermis.

Foot skin is the thickest on the body and ranges from 0.5 millimeters to an incredible 5 millimeters on the sole.

There are many skin problems to which the foot is especially susceptible.

Athlete's foot, a fungus infection called *tinea pedis,* is probably the most common skin disorder known to man. It's called athlete's foot for a very good reason. Athletes are particularly prone to this type of infection because of exposure to communal showers and locker rooms. You can get the infection from direct contact with an infected individual or from inanimate surfaces. It can occur in both sexes of all ages. Sweaty feet and ill-fitting shoes contribute to acquiring the disease. Most acute cases appear in hot weather.

The most common fungus organisms involved are *T. mentagrophytes* and *Monilia*. These organisms require dampness and darkness to flourish. Place a sweaty foot in a shoe and you create the perfect environment for the organisms to multiply. Excessive sweating causes tissue macerations, which in turn lowers the skin's normal surface acidity, which predisposes to infection.

The plantar surfaces of the foot in the arch and instep and between the toes are the favorite sites for an infection to develop. Itching, peeling of the skin, and cracking between the toes are the most common symptoms.

The primary eruption is a blister. Blisters break and dry out, which causes peeling of the skin. Often the skin is red and irritated. The skin between the toes will crack, become raw, and seep a clear, yellow, waterlike exudate that will form a crust as it dries.

The greatest danger presented by a fungus infection is that of secondary bacterial infection (pus) resulting from a crack in the skin. These infections must be treated professionally. Swelling, redness, pain, and pus are the symptoms to look for. This localized bacterial infection can go from a simple cellulitis to a generalized cellulitis characterized by red streaks running up the foot and leg. This can be followed by septicemia (blood poisoning).

When treating the problem, scrupulous personal hygiene must be employed. The feet should be washed twice daily with a mild soap. Avoid shoes that cause sweating. Wear clean socks that absorb moisture and change them twice a day. If you can, take your shoes and socks off and let your feet dry in the air, exposing your feet to sunlight. The ultraviolet rays of the sun are deadly to fungus organisms. There are excellent and generally safe medications with a fungicide that are available without prescription. Your pharmacist can recommend a good preparation. If the infection does not respond after a week or so of home treatment, consult a podiatrist. If there is any evidence of an infection, you should seek professional help. Your doctor can prescribe stronger medications that are not available over the counter.

Winter itch is a spontaneous cracking in the skin primarily involving the soles and the area of the big toe joint. It occurs most often in late fall and winter and affects mostly young people. It can be very uncomfortable and painful but does not represent any real danger. As with any crack in the skin, the great danger comes with the possibility of a bacterial infection.

Generally the cracking can be controlled with the application of a good lotion used for dry skin. In more severe cases Vaseline petroleum jelly is excellent. The condition usually corrects itself by the time spring rolls around.

Contact dermatitis (allergic reaction) is an acquired sensitivity to a continuous or interrupted external contact with a vegetable, mineral, or animal substance. Symptoms can run anywhere from a slight itching to severe blistering, drainage, and localized weeping. The distribution of the eruption is of extreme diagnostic importance. Initially the eruption involves only the areas exposed to the irritant. After a few weeks the eruption usually spreads. Treating this type of problem is almost always beyond the individual's own capabilities.

Hyperhidrosis, excessive sweating, and *bromidrosis,* excessive foot odor, plague millions of people.

Hyperhidrosis is a functional disorder of the sweat glands in which there is an excessive amount of sweat excreted without any apparent exciting cause. Sweating regulates the body temperature and eliminates body wastes. Localized hyperhidrosis is usually due to local trophic nerve dysfunction. The skin of the feet is blanched and macerated, the stockings are moist, and the shoe is often stained and water soaked. Treatment consists of the use of mild antiseptics and astringents. Shoes and socks should be changed twice a day. Hygienic measures are extremely important. The feet should be washed thoroughly at least once a day with soap and warm water. Some commercially available foot powders are helpful. Stronger medications require a prescription.

Bromidrosis is a functional disorder characterized by sweat excretion that has an offensive, fetid odor. It is most commonly associated with hyperhidrosis but not always. The foul odor is the result of bacterial decomposition of the sweat. Treatment is much the same as in hyperhidrosis. Rubber-soled shoes and tennis-type shoes should be avoided. Shoes and socks should be changed frequently and good hygiene observed.

Corns and callouses are best discussed under problems with the bones, because the hard skin you know as the corn is really a symptom of a problem with the underlying bone.

The *hard corn, heloma dura,* is found chiefly on the outside of the little toe, the top of the lesser toes, and on the very ends of the lesser toes as well. A corn is a thickening of the outer horny layers of skin over a bony prominence. The skin is caught between two unyielding surfaces: the shoe on the outside and the bone on the inside. The shoe presses on the bone, thus irritating it. Nature attempts to protect the irritated part by accumulating hard skin. Unfortunately nature does such a good job that before long the protective layer of hard skin acts as an irritant to the bone also. A corn is caused by intermittent pressure and friction.

There is a very simple and permanent cure for corns: Don't wear shoes! In today's society, however, it is not a very practical solution. Since we must wear shoes, great care should be exercised in their selection. Shoes must fit properly. If they don't feel good when you try them on at the store, they're not going to feel any better later on. You should own several pairs of everyday shoes so that you are not in any one pair long enough to cause problems. Exercise care when you put on your hose so that there are no twists or folds in the toe area.

If you already have a corn, there are certain measures you can take to lessen your misery. Having your shoe "spot" stretched by the shoemaker will help considerably. Be prepared to leave your shoe overnight. Soaking your foot in warm water with a little Epsom salts will give temporary relief. Ordinary hand lotion can help soften the area. Do not attempt to cut the hard tissue away. Bathroom surgery is dangerous and can lead to serious infection. Many of the over-the-counter remedies contain acid and eat away not only the corn but the normal tissue as well.

A painful corn will cause you to walk improperly. This incorrect gait quickly leads to other foot and leg problems.

Treatment runs from periodic palliative measures, such as reducing the hard skin and padding the area, to surgical correction. There are a variety of surgical approaches to the problem of corns and none of them is greatly incapacitating.

The *soft corn, heloma molle,* most frequently occurs in the web between the fourth and fifth toes, but can occur between all of the toes. It, too, is caused by intermittent pressure and friction, except the skin is caught between two bones instead of the bone and the shoe. Poorly fitting, tight shoes is usually the cause.

Because the corn is between the toes, it becomes macerated from sweat, and softens. It appears as a whitish or slightly yellow circumscribed overgrowth of the skin. Soft corns can become infected easily due to their unique location. Treatment is both palliative and surgical. Corn pads offer only temporary relief.

Hammertoe describes a clawing of the lesser toes with a resulting hard corn on the top of the toes and sometimes on the end of the toes. Improperly fitting shoes and/or arthritis are causative factors. Treatment consists of properly fit shoes, reduction of the painful corn, and padding.

A corn under the nail, *subungual heloma,* is not as common as the hard and soft varieties. It usually occurs under the first nail plate. Sometimes the corn is thick enough to lift and separate the nail from the nail bed. Pain is caused from pressure. As little pressure as that from the bedclothes can bring tears to the eyes. More often than not this type of corn is caused by one particular pair of shoes. If the culprit can be found and discarded in time, professional treatment may not be necessary.

A callous, *tyloma,* is a large mass of thickened skin on the bottom of the foot. The lesion is thick in the center and gradually tapers, becoming thin at the edges. There is no sharp line of demarcation between the callous and the normal skin. Close examination will reveal that the normal skin lines run through the entire growth even at the thick center area. Microscopically they are the same as a corn. The simple differentiation between the two is that corns involve toes and callouses occur on the bottom of the foot.

They are due to intermittent, excessive pressure and friction on a weight-bearing bone, often from poorly fitting shoes. Areas involved can be the metatarsal heads, heel, the plantar surface of the base of the fifth metatarsal, and under the first toe.

Symptoms of a callous run anywhere from a mild burning sensation to an excruciating pain from the slightest pressure. The pain is greater from direct pressure than from the sides.

Foot soaks, moleskin applied over the area, foam-rubber inserts, and keeping footgear in good order will give temporary relief.

Professional evaluation can determine the cause. Palliative measures such as cutting the tissue away and padding should be left to the podiatrist. It should be remembered that this type of treatment must be done periodically, as it affords only temporary relief. Treatment needs to be directed toward correcting imbalance and improving foot function. Orthotics can correct the biomechanical imbalance. Surgical correction involves bone.

Seed corns, *heloma miliare,* are very small, circumscribed growths, usually multiple, occurring on the bottom of the foot frequently in the heel area. They are rarely painful unless there are a great number of lesions present.

A *wart, verruca,* is a benign tumor involving the skin and is thought to be caused by a virus. They occur as single lesions or in a multiple form, and often spread from one part of the foot to the other. They occur in young people anywhere on the foot, but rarely on weight-bearing surfaces. Warts are normally very clearly circumscribed, and the skin lines go around the lesion rather than through it, as in the case of a callous. The dark spots that often appear are caused by small vessels breaking. They hurt from lateral pressure, as in a pinching action. The center of a wart is spongy, pale, and furrowed. The center of a callous is very hard. If a callous is misdiagnosed as a wart and excised, a painful scar can result.

On occasion warts will disappear spontaneously without any treatment. There are numerous methods of treatment for warts, which suggests that no treatment is infallible. X-ray therapy, cauterization, application of solidified carbon dioxide (dry ice), and ultrasound treatment have all been used with some success. Even hypnotherapy has been used successfully. Two popular methods of treatment are the application of an acid and surgical excision. Commercially available acid preparations can be dangerous. Excision can be accomplished with a surgical blade or a laser beam. Careless home treatment can lead to serious infection.

A *nevus* is a benign tumor involving skin: the common mole. They rarely present a problem unless found on a weight-bearing surface. A nevus should be watched carefully for any change in color or size, which can suggest malignancy.

A *malignant melanoma* is an adult skin tumor and one of the most virulent forms of skin cancer. It can arise out of the harmless nevus, can be flat or raised, small or large, and any color from red to brown to black. It can occur under the toenail as well. Any suspicious growth should be presented to your doctor for examination. Early detection is the key. Treatment consists of wide excision of the entire lesion and some of the surrounding skin. In some cases removal of the regional lymph nodes is required. Radiation treatment is generally of no value.

An *epidermal cyst* is an encapsulated mass filled with cheeselike material. It can vary in size from 0.5 to 3.0 centimeters and usually occurs on the bottom of the foot. These are painful only when a weight-bearing area is involved. On occasion they degenerate and become infected. A diagnosis is made by palpating a freely movable, circumscribed, subdermal mass of medium hardness. Treatment consists of surgical excision.

Although *ulcers* clearly involve the skin, they are discussed in detail in "Common Foot Problems Involving the Blood Vessels."

Keloid is the technical name given to enlarged, thickened, dermal fibrous tissue that forms after the skin is incised, whether surgically or from accidental laceration. The thickened scars tend to run in families. People with darker skin are more prone to keloid formation. The growths tend to recur after removal and can cause a great deal of difficulty if they form on a weight-bearing surface.

Kaposi's sarcoma frequently occurs in the feet as multiple, painful red or purple subcutaneous nodules. Because the tumor grows so slowly, wide surgical excision with skin graft and radiation therapy will often arrest the condition. It is very rare among blacks. It generally affects males and has a high incidence in young homosexual males with AIDS.

Psoriasis is a dominantly inherited disease that results in reddish or pink papules with scales that, when removed, often reveal pinpoint bleeding. It is a generalized disease but can affect the feet and toenails. Treatment is difficult.

There are several skin problems that commonly affect children.

Eczema is a term used to describe a dermatitis of unknown etiology. The lesions can be as simple as redness, swelling, and blistering or more complicated, with crusts from oozing and lichenification. Management is often a hit-or-miss affair. Eczemas have a strong hereditary influence. It comes and goes by itself and appears mainly on the flexor surfaces as oozing blisters and crusts, which result from scratching. Since itching is the major symptom, treatment is directed first toward relief and then toward the underlying cause that can be identified.

Lichen simplex, also called neurodermatitis, is characterized by a dry, thick, itchy, excoriated area. The skin is extremely itchy, and scratching usually results in a secondary bacterial infection. This condition is often associated with emotional upsets. Treatment is directed toward symptomatic relief and trying to resolve the patients emotional problems.

Pompholyx, also called dyshidrosis, presents as small recurring blisters on the palms and soles and is often associated with emotional stress. Relieve the stress, relieve the problem.

Peridigital dermatitis is a recurrent and persistent dermatitis that affects children's feet and is easy to confuse with common fungus infections. The skin is usually chronically scaling, with fissures that often involve the first toe. Steroid creams help.

Lichen planus is an inflammatory disease presenting as violet, flat-topped papules on the flexor surfaces of the skin. About 25 percent of the time the mucous membranes are involved as well. Steroid creams usually do the job.

Granuloma annulare affect female children more than males and appear as a donut-shaped pink area on the extensor surfaces of the extremities and the top of the foot. Most of the time it disappears spontaneously.

Bacterial infections can occur in the foot as primary problems. *Folliculitis* on the top of the foot and toes involves an infection of the hair follicle. On occasion the infection can become quite deep, and warm soaks, incision and drainage, and antibiotics will be required to resolve the problem.

Erysipelas is a streptococcal infection of the skin. It commonly occurs in newborn infants and in older children secondary to cracks in the web space. Blistering can occur, along with a high fever. Antibiotics are required for treatment.

Parasitic infestations, caused by larva migrans, that were once commonly seen in the southeastern United States in people who had contact with damp soil contaminated with feces is much less frequent now. Wearing shoes has reduced the incidence.

Scabies is a highly contagious skin disease caused by infestation with a mite. Itching is severe and worse at night. It occurs more commonly in the hands but can affect the feet. The characteristic lesion is a threadlike channel or burrow made by the female mite while laying her eggs. Specific creams are used to treat the problem, which can take months to resolve completely.

Common Foot Problems
Involving the Nails

The nails are the only part of the foot that anyone tries to make *more* beautiful than nature could manage. Women don't paint their heels or insteps. At most they use a moisturizer to bring back the smoothness and shine that nature intended.

Ah, but the nails. They are buffed, sprayed, and given colors God has yet to name. This does little harm, but it's ironic that so much time and effort is spent on beautifying the nails and so little on simple measures that could prevent the pain and suffering of a nail gone wrong.

The nails are appendages of the skin that serve the function of protecting the extremities of the toes from the nearly infinite number of threats presented by the world's sharp, heavy, and blunt objects. They are identifiable by the tenth week of fetal life and are necessary throughout life because, save perhaps for the eye and certain parts of the genital area, these extremities are the most sensitive parts of the human body.

To accomplish this protecting function, we are given a shield that is far more complex than an initial glance would indicate. The nail consists of a nail plate (the thing you call a nail), a nail bed, a nail fold, a cuticle, and a nail matrix. This last is composed of cells that grow the nail plate found under the skin and on top of the bone. It is nurtured by the blood vessels, the blood vessel end organs, and the nerve fibers. It generates the nail plate itself, an object consisting primarily of keratin and cystine.

Each of these components is vulnerable to disease, injury, and congenital malformation. Moreover, since the nails are cutaneous appendages (that is, they are related to the skin), they frequently reflect problems not directly related to the nails themselves but to the nearby skin.

Nonetheless one study of thousands of patients found that 94 percent of nail problems are due to local factors. Because nail problems often involve infection, the price for ignoring or mismedicating a problem usually comes due far more quickly than does a similar error with other foot problems. And the difficulty of treating such problems increases geometrically with the length of time for which the problem is ignored.

What You Should Be Doing to and for Your Nails

Toenails grow more slowly than fingernails, very approximately (depending on the person) about three inches a year. Thus every so often you have to cut your nails. This is usually where the trouble begins.

If you remember only one thing from this book, remember this: *Cut your nails straight across and even with the end of the toes.* No other single practice will do so much to avoid pain and expense.

Oh, sure, you say you'll do that and you knew it all along. However, think of the last time you trimmed your toenails. You knew that you should cut them straight and even began doing this. But then you noticed how classy they would look if you molded them to follow the contours of your toes. Then you decided to get rid of the sharp little corners that might snag your socks or stockings. Next you placed your newly trimmed toes in a narrow shoe. The blunt truth is that you followed to perfection the recipe for ingrown toenails.

Ideally you should not *cut* your nails at all. You should use an emery board and simply file them straight across. But we're realistic enough to know that most people will avail themselves of the ease of clippers or cutters. After all when was the last time you brushed your teeth after every meal as you know you should?

The cuticle also needs care, and this is best accomplished when the skin is softened by a shower or, better, a bath. However, do *not* cut your nails at this time. If you do, you'll find that drying shrinks the skin, pulling into the nail.

When the cuticle is wet, push it back gently with an orange stick (available at any pharmacy). Then, using a surgical-type scrub brush, scrub the nails well. This is important because your nails spend most of their lives in the altogether hostile environment of your shoes. How would *you* like to face the day in a black, sweaty, smelly, closed-off tunnel? The nail scrub is your only chance to undo the damage this life-style does.

Ingrowing toenail, called onychocryptosis, is an acute inflammatory condition of the soft tissue at the corner of the toenail, usually of the big toe.

There are three types of ingrown nails. The most common derives from a hook or spur resulting from improper cutting. This digs into the skin as the nail grows and refuses to let go. Less common is an inward distortion of the nail plate. Only about a quarter of all cases of ingrowing nails involve a deformity of the nail plate.

Under normal conditions the space between the nail margin and nail groove is about one millimeter. This space is sufficient to protect one from irritation under normal conditions. However, it is not sufficiently resistant to prevent overly tight shoes from exerting too-great downward pressure. This irritates the groove and causes a swelling that results in a thickening and a distortion of the nail lip—in short, an ingrowing nail.

You are probably familiar with the cycle. You notice it as the nail groove is cut by the nail margin, producing pain and the pus of secondary infection. In some cases "proud flesh" (granulation tissue) appears, bleeding, and retarding healing. If the bacterial infection is advanced, a foul odor accompanies the pain.

Congenitally thick nail lips predispose one to ingrown nails. This explains why infants who have never worn shoes develop the condition. Thick nail plates, whether due to congenital malformation or to any of numerous common fungus infections, are often the cause of ingrown nails.

If you are to avoid ingrown nails, it is crucial that you pay attention to shoe fit and shoe style. Avoid shoes with pointed toes. If either poor choice of shoe or foot abnormality causes a foot imbalance, take the necessary steps to correct the imbalance.

If you do get an ingrown toenail, soaking the affected foot in a mild solution of warm Epsom salts will help. Do *not* follow the old wives' solution of cutting a V in the nail plate. This will not help and may create a secondary bacterial infection.

In all but the mildest cases of ingrown toenails, you should look to professional care. If there is secondary infection, it must be taken care of immediately. There are a number of operative techniques that take care of the problem on the first try 85 percent of the time and that can be repeated should the infection recur.

Incurvated nail, also called an involuted nail, accounts for about a quarter of all ingrown-nail cases. An incurvated nail is essentially a deformity of the nail plate or bed or both. Its hallmark is an inward curving of the nail toward the end of the toe. Often the incurvation is a result of a deformation of the underlying bone, and both problems must be addressed. In any case professional attention is always required when a nail becomes incurvated.

Fungus infections of the nails, called onychomycosis, ringworm, and tinea unguis, are the most common of all inflammatory conditions involving the nails.

Fungi are parasites. They usually begin their assault on the outside of the nail and work their way into the nail root. They turn the nail dry, lusterless, and scaly, rendering the plate streaked and raised from the nail bed. They cause the nail plate to accumulate masses of dead skin and discolor the nail with brownish and yellow streaks. It is often the case that a fungus will remain on one nail for a long period and then suddenly spread to other nails.

Initial diagnosis is made by clinical observation, after which microscopic examination determines the specific organismic culprit. The disease becomes more common as we age, though it is far from unknown in children.

Fungi are notoriously difficult to treat. Treatment, which can take a very long time, ranges from systemic chemotherapy (taken orally) to the local application of topical drugs to the nail bed. Often the nail plate must be removed surgically. In severe cases infected shoes and socks must be discarded.

Onychia is an inflammation of the matrix (the cells that grow the nail plates). While it can involve any or all toes, it usually affects the great toe. When more than one nail is involved, the podiatrist will suspect a systemic cause, such as syphilis, tuberculosis, or an inflammatory skin disease.

However, onychia is ubiquitous. It can follow improper cutting of the nail or traumatic injury to the nail, such as that caused by a heavy object falling on the toe. It can even follow a localized trauma from shoe pressure and resulting secondary infection.

Onychia usually causes a loosening of the nail plate from its attachment and sometimes a shedding of the nail. The toe becomes red and swollen, and even light pressure can cause intense, throbbing pain.

Pressure must be relieved by establishing drainage, usually by complete removal of the nail plate. Once the acute symptoms and infection have been dealt with, attention can be directed toward the causes, whether they be local or systemic. Local germicides and fungicides are sometimes helpful.

Paronychia is essentially the same as onychia, but the side of the toe (the nail groove) is involved. Treatment is virtually identical to that for onychia.

Club nail, onychauxis, is a general term for a thickening of the nail plate over its entire area. It is usually caused by trauma, but tight shoes can predispose one to the condition. Syphilis, ichthyosis, and peripheral neuritis can also play a role in its genesis. It can occur on all the nails except the first, but the fifth toe is the most frequently involved. It is usually seen in older patients. When systemic involvement can be ruled out, general palliative care (that is, periodic reductions of the nails) usually suffice to control the situation. Surgical excision is rarely required.

Ram's horn nail, onychogryposis, differs from club nail primarily in that the nail plate, aside from being very thick, ultimately takes the form of a ram's horn. Poor hygiene and repeated trauma predispose to the affliction, and formerly it was found most frequently in men who attended horses. Today it is found most frequently in derelicts. It favors the first toe, but can affect any toe. Treatment is the same as that for club nail, and control is maintained by keeping the nails short.

Atrophy of the nails, onychatrophia, is defined as a condition in which the nails become smaller, thinner, and softer, frequently falling off altogether. Trauma or infection causes the cells that grow the nail (the matrix) to become malnourished. If the cause is systemic (an endocrine imbalance, for example) local treatment is worthless. Thus cause must be ascertained before treatment can be begun. Auxiliary local treatment consists of protection of the affected area from irritation, careful cutting of the nails, and sometimes an application of an ointment dressing.

Splitting of the nails, onychorrhexis, is characterized by a spontaneous longitudal splitting of the nail. It can vary in severity from a slight irregularity to a nail-deep splitting. Found mostly in older patients, it can affect even the young when it is symptomatic of eczema, psoriasis, or trophic conditions of the feet. Vitamins A and D are sometimes therapeutically helpful.

The appearance of *white spots in the nail plate,* leukonychia, can be congenital or subsequently acquired. In very rare cases the entire nail may be white. This condition is potentiated by a trauma that permitted air to enter between the nail plate and nail bed. It is not serious, which is good, since treatment leaves much to be desired.

Beau's lines are transverse lines that give the nail a wavy appearance. They begin at the base and grow forward. The transverse lines are due to sudden interruption of the functioning of the matrix cells that grow the nail. These irregular growth patterns are common side effects of infectious diseases and very high fevers. Treatment is rarely necessary, as the problem grows out naturally.

Spoon nails (koilonychia), and *anonychia* are relatively rare conditions. In the former the nail assumes a concave shape, while in the latter, which is congenital, the nail is missing completely.

Pterygium is not an extinct flying dinosaur but an overgrowth of cuticle that is easily rectified by trimming. Poor hygiene predisposes to this condition.

A *blood clot under the nail* is called a subungual hematoma. You've all had this. A trauma, such as smacking your toe into the bedpost, causes the toe to bleed under the nail. The nail becomes discolored from the blood underneath it and the pain is intense. In severe cases a hole is carefully drilled in the nail to permit drainage and reduce pressure. Vitamin C deficiency can also cause this problem. Whatever the cause, care must be taken to prevent a secondary bacterial infection.

Polyonychia refers to the presence of more than one nail on a toe. If you have polyonychia, you have already seen a podiatrist.

Psoriasis of the nail is characterized by a pitting of the nail plate and an onycholysis in which the nail plate has become separated from the nail bed. It is often an accompaniment to psoriatic arthritis. Because the nail often turns yellow, this malady can be confused with a fungus infection.

Psoriasis of the nail can present several additional problems. It can cause warts to grow very close to the nail. These facilitate diagnosis by providing tiny bleeding points that are easily identified. On some, fortunately very rare, occasions a malignant melanoma can occur under the nail plate.

There are many other psoriatic manifestations that, like a melanoma, require professional attention. Most are benign, but are difficult to identify. Benign fibroma, benign bone lesions (which occur mostly in children), and subungual exostosis are examples.

Glomus tumors, which appear as small, bluish-red lesions under the nail plate lying in the nail bed, can be exquisitely painful. They are discussed in greater detail in the section on problems involving the fat, fascia, and tendons.

Common Foot Problems
Involving the Fat,
Fascia, and Tendons

If you're like most Americans, you've probably spent more time than you'd like to admit thinking about fat—fat on your stomach, fat on your thighs, fat on all those places you wish you didn't have fat. Surprise: Guess where else you have fat? That's right, on your feet.

Actually this is a good thing. Fat is nature's cushion. If the feet had no fat all, weight bearing down on them would cause problems you don't even want to think about.

However, what works well most of the time can break down occasionally, and when it does, it hurts.

The good news is that problems with fat on the feet are very rarely life-threatening. The bad news is that, while not life-threatening, there are a lot of problems that can involve the foot's fat cells and associated fascia and tendon material.

Lipoma is the problem that is both the most common and the least often in need of treatment. A lipoma is simply a mass of fat cells that forms just beneath the skin and is, therefore, usually well defined and easily observed. Because lipoma can arise in areas otherwise without fat, altering the profile of the foot, it can be frightening. If you find that you have this, or any other tumor, you should see your doctor. If, as is most likely, the problem is a lipoma, he will assure you that there is nothing to worry about. Unless the lipoma is unusually large, no treatment will be required.

Giant-cell tumor is an even bigger bluffer than the lipoma. It scares its victim, usually a young person, half to death by growing to resemble a small planet and then is exposed by the doctor as merely a benign annoyance (though one that requires some professional treatment).

Xanthoma sounds like the bad guy in one of those "attack of the space aliens" movies. This looks like the bad guy in one of those "attack of the space alien" movies. But, just like in the movies, the good guys win. Like any self-respecting alien, the xanthoma is well encapsulated and fibroid, perfect for attacking your foot's tendon sheaths. Needless to say, it is filled with a truly disgusting, thick, brownish fluid. This ooze can be drained with a special needle made just for this purpose.

A *fibroma* is a tumor of the connective tissue. While fibromas can be found in any part of the foot, they most commonly attack the back of the heel and the top of the foot. Unlike our alien friend, they grow very slowly and rarely need treatment unless they are in locations causing pain. When this is the case, they are easily excised and rarely recur.

A *glomus tumor* is made up of convoluted blood vessels. If you have the GTs, you know it. Here we're talking real pain. The fact that a GT is benign makes it less frightening, but no less painful. It works like this: Usually blood goes from an artery to a vein through a route of microscopic capillaries. However, in certain areas of the skin of the toes, God left out the capillaries and substituted something called glomus cells. In all of the people most of the time and some of the people all of the time this all works fine and we can concentrate on things even more fascinating than glomus cells. However, on occasion a small nodular mass can form from these cells, and then . . . whooooeee. Like a blister, a glomus tumor can cause an amazing amount of pain for such a small area. A tiny area of the foot experiences a very severe throbbing pain and secondary burning. A really clever glomus can locate itself under a nail. If you have one of these, you're reading this in a doctor's office. Fortunately, a bit of local anesthetic and a minor excision end the problem and the pain.

Bursitis is a word people tend to use to refer to any of a great number of maladies, but it is correctly used to refer to an inflammation of a normal anatomic bursa. The only normal anatomic bursa to be found in the foot is the one between the heel bone and the Achilles tendon. "Normal" means it's supposed to be there. Unfortunately the body occasionally builds bursa where there shouldn't be any, specifically in areas subjected to repeated pressure or irritation over a long period of time. The bunion joint of the first toe is the most common location of an abnormal bursa of the foot. Not only can this cause considerable pain, but it is often also accompanied by a bacterial infection that complicates the already painful situation. Perhaps more than any other foot problem, bursa are treated with the widest range of therapies, from home care to hospitalization and surgery (depending on the severity of the problem). If there is no infection and the pain is not too severe, removal of the source of irritation, protection of the area with pads, and warm soaks can cure the problem. If there is infection, you must seek professional help.

Ganglion, like so many foot problems, are benign but painful. They usually attack the side of the first toe, the top of the foot, and the outside of the fifth toe. They can become impressively large, causing increasing pain with increasing size. It used to be thought that aspirating these lesions would help, so some practitioners would smash them with a large book. It didn't work. Today we have nonpainful methods, but not ones you can use at home.

Dupuytren's contracture is a fibrous growth first discovered by Guillaume Dupuytren in 1832. If, as is usually the case, you get a

Dupuytren contracture on the palm of your hand, you'll have to read another book to find out what to do. Dupuytren's contracture occurs on the plantar aspect of your foot. These hard growths usually affect children and young adults. We're not sure why they appear or what causes them, but we do know that they are easy to excise and should be excised if they become large. When ignored, DC can lead to a loss of elasticity of the thick, fibrous band that runs on the bottom of the foot from the heel to the toe area, the plantar fascia.

Plantar fasciitis is a tenderness of the plantar fascia that becomes outright painful when the area is palpated. While not serious in and of itself, this should warn you of the possibility of one or another of the arch problems discussed in another chapter.

Tenosynovitis sounds like something that happens to someone who plays the net game for the first time, and indeed the pressure put on the foot by certain sports can cause tenosynovitis. More commonly the cause of this inflammation of the tendon and its sheath is the trauma of a home accident, like that resulting from a soup can falling on the foot. Infection of an area adjacent to a laceration spreads to the tendon and its sheath. If the resulting laceration gets infected, professional help is required. The podiatrist will first treat the infection and then offer such supportive measures as foot soaks, pads for shoes, and physiotherapy.

The good news is that malignant tumors of the soft tissue of the feet are quite rare. The better news is that they are often treated successfully with wide radical resection, skin grafting, and radiotherapy.

The most common types of malignant tumors of the soft tissue of the foot are fibrosarcoma, synovial cell sarcoma, and angiosarcoma (Kaposi's sarcoma).

Kaposi's sarcoma is increasing in frequency as AIDS (Acquired Immune Deficiency Syndrome) is increasing in frequency. Its first noticeable form is a painful red or yellow subcutaneous nodule that can become almost wartlike in appearance. This growth enlarges slowly and is treatable by the method described above.

Fortunately a *liposarcoma* is rarely found in the foot, for when it is, amputation is indicated. It is not always easy, however, to tell a liposarcoma from the more common lipoma, so care must be taken in diagnosis.

A *clear-cell sarcoma* is a malignant tumor that occurs in the Achilles tendon and the plantar fascia. It is a painless swelling found usually in young adults. It is very difficult to diagnose and can be innocently excised as a benign mass, only to be discovered to be cancerous when examined by the pathologist.

Primary muscle tumors, both benign and malignant, are found in the foot so rarely that they do not require discussion here.

Finally, there are four well-defined fascial compartments in the lower leg. Any one of a number of compartment syndromes can occur when the muscular contents of a compartment swell beyond the elastic limits of the surrounding fascia. Problems of this sort are common among runners and are discussed in the chapter on running.

Common Foot Problems
Involving the Blood Vessels

Neither the vascular system of the foot nor the task it performs is terribly complicated. The role of the arteries and veins is simply to bring clean, oxygenated, nutrient-rich blood to the foot and to take dirty, depleted blood back to the heart for restoration.

The names of the arteries and veins that accomplish this are complicated. For example, the primary sources of arterial supply are the anterior and posterior tibial arteries and the two terminal branches of the popliteal artery. The former run down the front and back of the leg, respectively, with the posterior tibial artery entering the foot just behind and beneath the inside ankle bone called the medial malleolus.

All of these arteries branch into smaller and smaller vessels that complete the transportation of the blood from the heart to the farthest reaches of the toes. The veins of the leg and foot, which are charged with the job of getting the blood back to the heart, are divided into two groups: the superficial and the deep. The veins are able to accomplish this task because they are fitted with mechanisms that prevent retrograde flow of the blood, which would, of course, poison the system and render life impossible.

The superficial group of veins lie just beneath the skin (therefore their name), while the veins of the deep group follow the arteries. Just as the arteries decrease in size as they journey away from the heart, the veins increase in size as they journey toward the heart.

Venous thrombosis is one of many problems concerned with a blockage of blood flow and refers to a clot, usually in one of the deep veins of the foot, that causes an impairment of the body's ability to return blood to the heart. Often occurring after a long period of inactivity, such as prolonged bed rest while recuperating from an illness, or even an extended period of sitting, venous thrombosis is known to be associated with various serious disease processes.

The most common initial sign that we are dealing with a thrombosis is a pain and tightness in the calf that are moderate in degree and constantly present. These symptoms will increase with walking, and running will be nearly impossible. The calf will often swell and the foot will become cyanotic in color. Invariably palpation will elicit pain.

Both diagnosis and treatment are less severe than the seriousness of the problem would lead one to believe. Various noninvasive techniques are utilized to identify the thrombosis, and therapy usually consists of resting with the legs raised. The person is told to move his foot through its full range of motion and to engage in activity that strengthens the pumping action required to clear the affected area and get the blood back on its way to the heart. On occasion blood thinners, such as heparin, are used, and the constellation of aforementioned conservative techniques is usually successful.

Chronic venous insufficiency simply describes problems involving obstruction of the venous outflow of the foot. Whether caused by a growth or a diseased induced breakdown of a valve, the end result is a greatly reduced venous blood return to the heart.

The symptoms in such cases are clear-cut. A chronic swelling of the leg and a dark brown discoloration is often coupled with both infection and ulceration, particularly stasis ulceration inside the ankle bone (medial malleolus).

As with other venous dysfunctions, the primary therapy consists of elevation of the leg. Elastic support hose and an Unna's boot often reduce pain by acting as a soft cast providing compression dressings to the ulcerated area.

When a foot becomes ischemic, the interruption of the arterial blood supply alerts the practitioner to the likelihood of *arterial occlusive disease*. Diagnosis and therapy must first consider whether the disease is acute or chronic, whether it is fast or slow in its development, and whether the symptoms appear at a slower or faster rate than that at which the disease progresses. If the damage is proceeding with haste, immediate action must be taken. If, on the other hand, the disease is progressing slowly, the body can often build substitute vessels to provide a collateral circulation to the area involved.

Arterial embolism is a dramatic disorder that can require amputation. It is characterized by a sudden blockage by an embolism that journeys down smaller and smaller vessels until it enters one from which it cannot exit. There are two basic types of emboli: the macroembolus, which, as its name implies, is large, ranging from 5 to 10 or more millimeters in diameter. Smaller, but still potent, is the microembolus.

Embolisms begin when cardiac irregularity following myocardial infarction of the left ventricle (heart attack) wall dislodge clots of dead heart muscle. Larger emboli become trapped in vessels of decreasing size, usually at a point of bifurcation. The most common areas in which such emboli come to rest are the terminations of the aortic, common iliac, common femoral, and popliteal arteries.

As soon as the embolism becomes lodged, the foot is threatened. There is no chance that the incident will be missed. The onset of ischemia is very rapid. The patient will notice pallor (paleness), partial paralysis of the foot, and will experience excruciating pain. There will be an absence of pulses distal to the clot, and the lack of oxygen to the area will cause an ischemic myositis. Often the ankle joint will lock and resist any attempt to move it. On occasion the patient presents a cyanosed toe representing "blue-toe syndrome."

This is rigor mortis. When this occurs, the foot is dead. While the average time for this to occur is about six hours, neither a three- nor a twelve-hour period is unknown. The ability of collateral circulation to feed the area determines the precise time that will have to pass before rigor mortis sets in.

The more distal the embolis, the greater the chance of irreparable harm, with the highest rate of limb loss being associated with an embolus of the popliteal artery.

With microemboli the symptoms are less dramatic, but loss of toes or foot are not-unknown results of these small clots. This can happen when emboli of the walls of the larger arteries cause embarrassment of the circulation of one or two toes (the number dependent on whether an embolism at a point of bifurcation blocks the route to one or two digits).

Arteriosclerosis obliterans is the most common of the chronic obliterative arterial diseases. It is usually found in males, the elderly, and people with diabetes.

Because arteriosclerosis obliterans is a disease in which the lumen, the interior of the vessel, is gradually reduced in size and less and less capable of accepting blood and the nourishment it offers, smoking is deadly for the victim of this disease. The vasoconstrictor effect of smoking is so profound that the lowering of the skin temperature owing to one cigarette can be measured up to six hours after the cigarette is smoked! And smoking does not merely exacerbate the disease once one has it; the smoker is five times as likely to get arteriosclerotic lesions as is the nonsmoker.

Often the first sign of the disease is an intermittent claudication characterized by calf pain after only a short bit of walking. The pain is such that the patient must rest and rub his calf before he can resume walking. His foot and toe will feel cold and appear blanched; often a "pins and needles" sensation accompanies the pain.

The end result is a complete blockage of the vessels with a resultant ulceration and gangrene. The latter, which is simply the death of tissue, usually occurs in the toes. This is often accompanied by changes in nail development, cessation of hair growth, and inhumanly shiny skin.

When conservative treatment is possible, it is long-term. Above all the patient must be taught, and must learn, the cause and nature of the disease and must be persuaded to accept the changes these demand. Tobacco is strictly forbidden; continued smoking for one with this disease is suicide. A reduction of weight is strongly advised, if only to reduce the load on the feet.

All patients, but especially diabetics, are taught to carefully examine their feet daily. Shoes that are well-fitted but sufficiently large to avoid irritation are a must, and thicker socks are strongly recommended. All in all, the diseases discussed here stem from poor health habits and result in a reduction of life's pleasures.

Thromboangiitis obliterans, also known as Buerger's disease, is not nearly as common as arteriosclerosis obliterans. While it, too, occurs most often in males, in this case it is males under forty. The cause of the disease is unknown. It is known, through microscopic study, that it affects the smaller arteries and arterioles and that it is usually accompanied by an obstructive thrombus. Again, tobacco plays a villainous role in this disease.

An immediate diagnostic element permitting us to distinguish this disease from arteriosclerosis obliterans is the cramping of the foot instead of the calf. Ulceration and gangrene can occur as the disease progresses. Treatment consists of absolute avoidance of tobacco, and supportive measures. Vasodilators are usually not effective.

The symptomatology of *Raynaud's phenomenon* is a function of the temperature in which the patient finds himself: cold causes episodic vasoconstriction of the smaller arteries of the hands and feet. In acute attacks the changes of skin color can be quite dramatic. Extreme pallor is followed by blue discoloration and, finally, a red flush.

It is termed *Raynaud's disease* when the condition is primary, without any causal disease and is found almost solely in young adult females. It shows no favoritism with respect to ethnic group.

Raynaud's can affect any limb and often alters nail growth. It is found in the early stages of lupus erythematosus and other serious collagen disturbances, but most cases of Raynaud's are not connected with lupus.

While medications such as guanethidine and phenoxybenzamine are often helpful, the primary therapy is avoidance of cold.

Diabetes is not of course a vascular disease. However, arteriosclerosis obliterans usually accompanies long-term diabetes. In an irony far from unknown in medicine, success at defeating the most serious effects of a disease have resulted in an increase in effects that are less serious, but serious nonetheless.

At one time coma and death were such common accompaniments of diabetes that diabetic ulcers and other side effects of compromised circulation did not have as much time to develop.

The atherosclerotic lesions that block the vessels of diabetics are identical with those that afflict nondiabetics, save for their arriving at a much earlier age and their greater likelihood of occurring in the legs and feet.

This disease often calcifies the vessel walls, with a resulting rigidity of the arteries. In nondiabetics such a reduction in circulatory efficiency is often complemented by the body's ability to build a collateral circulation to the affected part. The diabetic body is not capable of doing this.

Diabetics face a host of additional problems of the vessels. Microangiopathy is a common disorder of the small vessels that, like neuropathies, decrease sensitivity and permit accidents that exacerbate the problems already present. The combination of a circulatory system damaged by arterial occlusion and diabetic neuropathy often cause such a lack of sensitivity that the diabetic fails to notice symptoms that would lead others to get help. As a result when the practitioner does finally get to see the diabetic, the disease is well advanced.

Diabetic ulcers, which are discussed at greater length in the chapter on the diabetic foot, are classified by degree of severity, from least pathological to most severe.

A grade-zero ulcer is not open, but has thickened keratoses that increase the potential for ulceration. A grade-one involves only the skin, while a grade-two is found in tendons and joint capsules. A grade-three involves bone, often with osteomyelitis. Grades four and five both involve gangrene, with the former localized and the latter destroying a major section of the foot.

It is infinitely better to prevent ulcers than to attempt to treat them once they develop. This is a simple procedure (or as simple as diabetes ever allows) with patients having grade-zero ulceration. Patient education, proper footgear, daily inspection of the feet, and frequent visits to the podiatrist for evaluation and treatment often permit a grade-zero patient to avoid grade-one ulceration. In addition underlying arterial occlusive disease can be greatly reduced by a cessation of smoking and an appropriate exercise program.

Often ulcerations, even in a grade-one patient, become infected, with more than one type of microorganism doing the damage. Identification of the microorganisms and treatment with the indicated antibiotic usually keep serious problems of infection at bay.

A grade-one foot requires debridement of the dead tissues and the elimination of pressure with appropriate dressings, while a grade-two may require skin grafts. A grade-three foot with osteomyelitis requires aggressive and long-term antibiotic treatment, while grade four usually requires partial amputation. Both podiatrist and patient often opt for the minimal amputation possible (for example, a toe or transmetatarsal). Sometimes this is sufficient; other times it fails and a grade-five foot develops, requiring amputation well above the infected area.

There are various types of *ulcers* in addition to diabetic ulcers. For example *trophic ulcers* occur in association with neurological disease processes. As with diabetic ulcers, these are usually the result of an insensitivity that is incapable of perceiving localized irritation.

Immersion foot, a malady first identified and named during World War II, is caused by long periods of immersion in cold water and the decrease in the arterial blood supply to the foot that it engenders. Treatment is nearly always successful and consists of elevation, cooling of the extremity, and antibiotics.

Trench foot is another cost of war. It is a cold injury ensuing from prolonged periods without walking and subzero temperatures, an environment perfectly presented by a foxhole. Pain, loss of feeling, and reduction of motion are complemented by a blanching and a blue discoloration, followed by blister formation. At its worst, trench foot can result in gangrene. Immediate therapy includes removal of the boot, massage of the skin, and a change of socks. When medical facilities are available, treatment resembling that for immersion foot is usually successful.

Chilblain, also called pernio, is a common affliction caused by repeated exposure of bare skin to wet, wind, and cold. It is identifiable by the skin's becoming red, itchy, and swollen.

Frostbite is an actual localized freezing of the outer tissues of the body. It most commonly attacks the face, hands, and feet. When hypothermia, the cooling of the body's deep inner core, is also present, the dangers are very great.

Damaged tissue freezes readily, and frostbite presents a constant threat to skiers, mountain climbers, and others likely to be injured at high altitudes. But even on the streets of northern cities alcoholics and homeless people often succumb to frostbite and hypothermia.

It is not merely the cold but also the heights endured by skiers and mountain climbers that renders these individuals susceptible to frostbite. At altitudes above six thousand meters the air offers less oxygen for nourishment of the tissues. In response to the chronic hypoxia conditions, the body produces an excess of red blood cells. This in turn causes the blood to become viscous and sluggish. It's as if you added some oil to the gas in your gas tank. With the blood in this state the formation of small emboli in the arteries of the limbs and thrombi in the leg veins becomes an increasing likelihood.

When the fluid in a cell freezes, the cell nucleus breaks down and the cell dies. This, incidentally, is why cryonics, the attempt to freeze dying individuals until the time that we have a cure for their diseases, is doomed for the foreseeable future; the freezing and unfreezing process destroys them from within.

Deep frostbite kills tissue and nerve and causes a loss of the sensations of pain and cold that protect us. Often the first sign noticed by one affected with frostbite is a blistering and blue mottling of the skin. External frozen tissue feels solid, and a deeply frozen limb feels tight and is difficult to move.

If you notice these symptoms developing, you must rest and elevate the affected limb, and you *must* keep it clean. Otherwise, infection is certain to develop.

When the situation permits, a rewarmed and thawed climber should be carried down the mountain. However, if shelter is available, it should be utilized. Fast rewarming is less dangerous than slow, but the frostbitten area should never be thawed over an open flame. Cooking is more likely to happen than healing!

Ideally the limb should be immersed for twenty to forty minutes in water that is 42 degrees centigrade. Hotter water will cause further damage, and colder will do little to thaw the area. Thawing must continue until the flesh is warmed, soft, pliable, and flush red. Unfortunately the pain of this process is severe, but temporary pain is preferable to loss of limb. As always, care must be taken to keep the part clean in order to prevent infection.

Superficial frostbite, which is much more common, damages only surface cells. The frozen tissue becomes white and waxy, but it is soft and pliable when pressed. The skin tingles and hurts. While this is no one's idea of pleasant, it is a sign that there has not been nerve damage. Therefore you can jump up and down, wiggle your toes, and flex your ankles to increase circulation. You should not, however, rub your skin vigorously, for this increases the chance that the skin will break, opening the area to infection from without. Never rub snow into the frozen area; on a microscopic level snow crystals are like glass and they affect the frozen area in much the same way as glass would. Do not cut or drain the blisters, which protect the underlying tissue, and keep it sterile. Proper treatment almost always enables one suffering from superficial frostbite to recover without any loss of tissue.

Under the extreme conditions encountered by the mountain climber, that which would be a small inconvenience at sea level becomes potentially lethal. As small a thing as a wrinkled sock does not merely cause irritation but interferes with the flow of blood. Tight boots cramp the mechanisms of circulation and introduce possibly lethal infections.

For all of the above reasons, it is crucial that if you are spending prolonged periods in snow, even at sea level, you have with you a pair of dry socks. If your feet feel very cold or lose sensation, immediately remove your boots, warm your feet, and put on the dry socks. The socks, by the way, can also serve as substitute gloves.

If you don't have dry socks, plastic bags make good vapor barriers that trap the warmth of the sweating foot. (Bootmakers have discovered this principle and now make plastic double-lined boots that are waterproof and resistant to the freezing that can crack leather in very cold temperatures.)

There are primarily congenital disorders in addition to diabetes that engender problems similar to those we have mentioned. *Hemophilia,* which became known as the "disease of royalty" in the days when no one cared about the many nonroyal people who had it, is a disorder of blood coagulation that is transmitted through the female but affects the male. Hemophilia is a rare disease that attacks fewer than one person in eight thousand.

The most common manifestation of the disease is a bleeding into the muscles and joints. Nearly all male hemophiliacs suffer some degree of muscle and joint damage by the time they reach maturity. The most commonly affected joints are, in descending order, those of the knees, elbows, ankles, shoulders, and hips. The small joints of the feet are usually involved only after trauma. In children the order of damage is somewhat altered, with the ankle being most commonly affected.

The first task in all cases of hemophiliac damage is the treatment of joint bleeding and replacement of missing blood-clotting factors. Then attention can be given to actual damage to the joints.

Pain in joints can be relieved by elastic bandages, though severe pain can require plaster-of-Paris casts and their ability to immobilize the joints in the most comfortable position that can be obtained. Isometric exercises should be started as soon as the acute symptoms subside in order that atrophy be avoided. Later, muscle-strengthening and range-of-motion exercises can be undertaken.

Diseases that alter the structure or the rate of production of the hemoglobin molecule of the blood are called *hemoglobinopathies*. The most common examples of hemoglobinopathies are sickle-cell diseases, sickle-cell trait, and hemoglobin SC disease.

Each of these disorders can cause both bone pathology and leg ulceration. In *sickle-cell disease* the majority of hemoglobin molecules is abnormal. This leads to the patient suffering from a multitude of problems and successive crises that eventually cause severe disability and decreased longevity.

In *sickle-cell trait,* less hemoglobin is impaired, and there is correspondingly less symptomatology. Patients with *hemoglobin SC disease* suffer abnormalities and symptoms falling somewhere between the other two maladies. All three are found primarily among blacks.

The name of these diseases comes from the crescentic shape of the involved red blood cells, a shape that permits them to become easily trapped in the microvessels. This trapping begins a feedback process in which a microcirculatory stasis causes a tissue hypoxia that in turn promotes further sickling. The end result of this vicious circle is tissue necrosis and bone infarcts. The infarcts of the small bones of the hands and feet produce a characteristic dactylitis that is called hand and foot disease. There is often a bilateral symmetry to soft-tissue swelling, but it is rare for both hands and feet to be involved at the same time.

As with so many of the diseases we have discussed in this chapter, sickle-cell syndromes usually include ulceration of the legs.

These are usually found on the medial and lateral aspect of the distal tibia and sometimes on the sole and dorsum of the foot.

Treatment of ulceration owing to sickle-cell diseases consists of wet-to-dry dressings and bed rest. Antibiotics are used to defend against infection, and elastic stockings are worn to enable the patient to avoid unnecessary trauma and pain.

Common Foot Problems
Involving the Nerves

While problems affecting the nerves of the foot are far from uncommon, diseases intrinsic to these nerves are rare. When the nerves of the feet are severely impaired, it is nearly always a sign of problems elsewhere, most seriously upper (brain) and lower (spinal column) neuron disease.

Differentiating between the two is the doctor's first task when he suspects that he is encountering neuron disease. In an example of diagnosis arrived at from symptoms far removed in location and nature from the disease generating those symptoms, the doctor will examine the gait of the person afflicted. Because upper and lower nerve diseases affect gait differently, the two can be differentiated on these grounds.

Upper neuron disease generates a narrowness in the base of the step in gait, and the body's weight is borne on the ball of the foot. Muscles are spastic, but there is no atrophy. Multiple sclerosis is the primary example of upper neuron disease affecting the feet.

Lower neuron disease, on the other hand, broadens the base of the step in gait and causes muscular flaccidity and atrophy. This is seen in anterior poliomyelitis, a disease now rare, thanks to the Salk and Sabin vaccines.

You might think that neurological disorders are inevitably associated with pain. Certain nerve disorders can cause intense pain, although it is often true that the symptom indicating the disorder is numbness or insensitivity.

Causalgia, for example, is characterized by severe local pain and burning, often accompanied by secondary redness and blister formation. It results from the incorporation of a nerve into a surgical or postfracture scar. Gunshot wounds or other direct trauma are usually the initiating cause.

While the pain from causalgia often marks the precise spot of the nerve lesion that is causing it, it can also be the result of the "phantom pain" experienced by amputees. *Phantom pain* "occurs" in an area of the body that has been amputated. Obviously this cannot be the true source of the pain, though the experience of pain is indistinguishable from that of an injury to a still-viable limb.

Phantom pain is still far from entirely understood, but it is clear that living nerves are continuing to receive signals identical to those that would be sent by living tissue and are forwarding these signals to the brain.

Where, not long ago, we had to watch helplessly as patients who had already suffered the trauma of amputation were forced to endure endless phantom pain, in recent years methods have been developed for alleviating it. Primary among these are whirlpool baths and motion exercise, which are far more effective than they sound, and direct injection of local anesthetic into the area at which the amputation has taken place. If this is not effective, surgical removal of all scar tissue will often reduce local pressure and the pain it generates. In recalcitrant cases a sympathectomy, the excision of the regional nerve supply responsible for relaying the pain signals, is performed.

It is sometimes the case that a general neuropathic disease far removed from the foot will "save" most of its symptomatic devastation for the foot. Such *neuropathic syndromes* are often found in patients with *severe diabetes*.

In such cases the initial symptom is not pain but an insensitivity in the peripheral nerves of the foot. However, because this insensitivity renders the patient unable to notice the sorts of infection-inducing events that the rest of us would notice and rectify, serious infections develop and run rampant before being discovered. This process is abetted by a deterioration of peripheral circulation and a resulting reduction of the body's ability to destroy the invading organisms.

It is crucial that the diabetic patient be educated to recognize the initial warning signs of neurological dysfunction. Often the first is a loss of the vibratory sense. A daily foot examination is the minimal requirement of a judicious approach to diabetes. Footgear should be examined for any flaw that could be the source of irritation. The feet themselves must, of course, also be examined daily. It is not uncommon to hear of a patient who stepped on a thumbtack and walked around for several days without noticing it; such is the degree of insensitivity. Unfair as it may seem, the same insensitivity that permits this, and an ensuing infection, to occur also permits the infection and its spread to areas that are still sensitive and still capable of experiencing acute pain. (Turn back to the chapter on the diabetic foot for further information.)

Syphilitic neuropathy and its effects on the feet are mercifully far less common than they were in the days before antibiotics reduced syphilis from a major killer of human beings to "merely" a serious, but treatable disease. Where once syphilis routinely resulted in destruction of the knee joint, today it is stopped in its tracks in its early stages by a bit of penicillin.

The majority of nerve disorders encountered by the foot doctor are those resulting not from disease but from crush injuries, lacerations, and thermal injuries, both hot and cold, such as those resulting from gunshots.

To understand how such traumata affect the body, it is necessary to have at least a simplified picture of the peripheral nerve.

The nerve itself is composed of a connective-tissue sheath called the epineurium. These are enclosed in surrounding bundles of nerve fibers called funiculi. Each of these bundles is surrounded by its own sheath of perineurium. Finally these bundles are separated by connective tissue known as the endoneurium.

When encountering a patient with a *traumatic injury to the nerve,* the physician's first task is to assess the degree of injury to the axon. In a first-degree injury there is what is referred to as a conduction deficit without axonal interruption, or more simply stated, no anatomical tear to any of the nerve structures.

In a second-degree injury the axon is severed without a breaching of the endoneurium. More serious is a third-degree disintegration of the axon with an accompanying disorganization of the internal structure of the funiculi. Most serious, a fourth-degree nerve injury is an axonal rupture with funicular and perineurial disruption.

Not all nerve problems of the feet are as serious as those discussed to this point. With an increasing emphasis on physical fitness, for example, we see greatly increased numbers of cases of *compression neuropathies.*

Remember when you thought, If everyone else is jogging, why not me? Remember when images out of the diet-soda ads, images of women so thin you could see through them and men chiseled out of stone running toward each other on a beach of snow-white sand, convinced you that only health and beauty lay ahead on the long running trail? Probably compression neuropathy didn't play that big a role in your fantasies. Nonetheless that's when the specter of compression neuropathy loomed over your life.

The direct causes of compression neuropathy are many and inglorious. Direct trauma is the most obvious cause and the easiest to diagnose. But the stretching of a nerve or the compression of a neighboring nerve can have this same effect. More difficult to identify as culprit is the entrapment of a nerve passing through sites bounded by bone and ligament, bone and fascia, or fascia and fascia.

Indeed wherever two things are in close proximity in the foot, the compression of a nerve is a possibility, a potential just waiting for its owner to decide to jog.

Maladies such as these can be acute and of sudden occurrence or chronic and a long time a-comin'. The former are typically related to a specific event, a misstep or stepping on a rock, and are accompanied by edema and inflammation. The latter more often result from overuse, a tendency of the enthusiastic beginner and the obsessive (a type hardly unknown in jogging), and hypertrophy.

It should not be thought that, in real life, afflictions of the type discussed easily categorize themselves. Diagnosis is often as tedious for the doctor as the problem is painful for the patient. To a great extent this is a result of the fact that there is simply so much going on in the affected areas and so many possible causes of entrapment.

For example when a peripheral nerve exits deep soft-tissue planes and passes through layers of fascia, any of the many layers can serve as a vise to press on the nerve. Likewise when muscles are enlarged and forcibly contracted, the muscles themselves can do the entrapping. Not surprisingly, weight lifters and bodybuilders encounter this so often that they come to see it as a normal part of life.

Whatever the cause of a nerve injury, it is generally true that the degree of injury determines the likelihood of recovery and the degree of discomfort. We have all experienced transient nerve entrapment when, after crossing our legs or sitting in an awkward position, we have found that our leg has "fallen asleep." Your leg falls asleep because direct pressure on the peroneal nerve causes a transient paralysis that, as it is abating, can cause considerable pain different in feeling from any other. Fortunately as soon as circulation is restored, anesthesia, paralysis, and pain are gone and recede from memory. (One of the greatest gifts we have received from evolution is the inability to reexperience physical pain; imagine how awful it would be if the memory of the last time you smacked your toe against the bedpost hurt as much as the actual incident.)

Incidents such as the sleeping leg are minor. A more serious version can occur when an intoxicated person passes out (or falls asleep—the difference is real, but subtle) on his arm. This longer-term ischemia does not merely compress the nerve, it damages the epineural sheath. Similar injuries can damage nerves of the feet, and as you might guess, the longer the pressure causing the entrapment, the more serious the entrapment.

We can best understand the various forms of compressive nerve entrapment by examining each of the major nerves individually.

The sciatic nerve is the one that the nurse always tries to avoid when giving you an injection south of the border. Pressure on the lumbar root of the sciatic nerve, resulting from, say, a herniated disc, often results from a bending motion not seemingly different from one you've made a thousand times before. When you see a TV character or close relative bend over, try to stand up, and then go "Oooo . . . ," you may well be seeing the syndrome in action.

Worse yet is entrapment from muscular enlargement at the sciatic notch. This spot is particularly vulnerable because it is where the external rotator muscles of the hip can force the body into unnatural positions. (For this reason you should *not* do twisting sit-ups.)

While bending is the primary cause of sciatic problems, walkers, joggers, and runners do not escape. Vigorous movement of this sort can cause lumbar lordosis, a compression of the nerve against the sciatic notch.

Treatment for all of these problems tends to be conservative. Rest, nonsteroidal anti-inflammatory medications, and careful attention to correct walking, jogging, or running are usually all that is required for complete recovery. Recurrent events of this nature are usually owing to a too-speedy return to exercise done in the incorrect manner that caused the problem in the first place.

The *obturator nerve* permits motor function from the medial thigh to the knee. Bodybuilding and power lifting can, and often do, cause an entrapment that can be relieved by rest and medications of the sort mentioned above. However, getting a bodybuilder to take a rest is akin to asking an alcoholic to refrain from drinking, and obturator problems tend to last far longer than necessary.

Some nerve entrapments can cause a severe burning feeling. When, for example, the *lateral femoral cutaneous nerve,* which supplies sensation to the anterior and lateral thigh, becomes entrapped at the level of the inguinal ligament, a severe burning paresthesia can result. The fact that this can be seriously aggravated by merely carrying heavy objects in the pocket shows the role that leerage plays in many nerve problems. Fortunately this one nearly always responds to conservative treatment.

Entrapment of the *saphenous nerve,* which is a branch of the femoral nerve, interferes with the saphenous' normal function of supplying sensation to the medial sides of the knees, calf, and ankle. The burning sensation associated with entrapment between the fascia of the vastus medialis and the adductor magnus is usually the result of prolonged walking or standing and usually comes at night. It is neither uncommon nor serious.

The *peroneal nerves* are extensions of the sciatic nerve that take various paths to the foot. They are vulnerable to virtually all the problems discussed in this chapter and are encountered by bodybuilders, weight lifters, joggers, and runners, particularly the practitioners of these endeavors who believe that too much of a good thing is never enough. Compression and paresthesias in any of many areas between the knee and the foot is often due to pressure on the peroneal nerve, as are similar symptoms in the foot itself.

In addition to the usual conservative treatments of immediate and extended rest and (often) nonsteroidal drugs, heel lifts and lateral sole wedges can give immediate relief from symptoms (though the cause still requires healing time). When peroneal entrapment affects the top of the foot, it is crucial to wear shoes of adequate depth so as not to irritate the top of the foot. In such cases orthotics can be most helpful in giving support to the medial longitudinal arch. These inlays made from an impression of the feet can be transferred from shoe to shoe. In extreme cases steroid medications may be called into play.

The *posterior tibial nerve* runs beneath the flexor retinaculum and

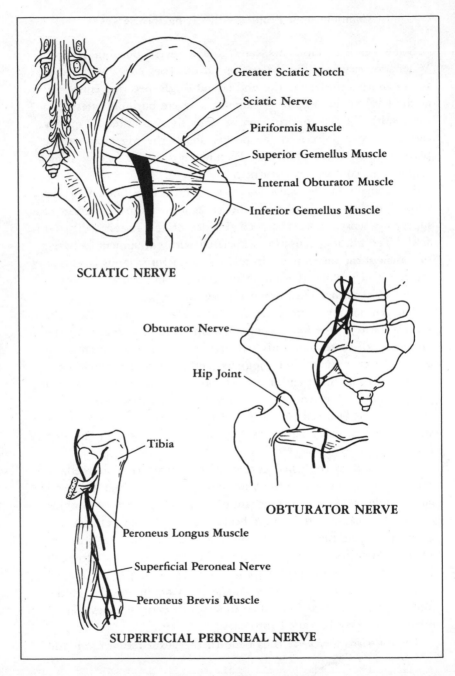

Greater Sciatic Notch

Sciatic Nerve

Piriformis Muscle

Superior Gemellus Muscle

Internal Obturator Muscle

Inferior Gemellus Muscle

SCIATIC NERVE

Obturator Nerve

Hip Joint

OBTURATOR NERVE

Tibia

Peroneus Longus Muscle

Superficial Peroneal Nerve

Peroneus Brevis Muscle

SUPERFICIAL PERONEAL NERVE

SUPERFICIAL PERONEAL NERVE

- Common Peroneal Nerve
- Peroneus Longus Muscle
- Superficial Peroneal Nerve
- Tibia
- Deep Peroneal Nerve

DEEP PERONEAL NERVE

- Deep Peroneal Nerve
- Inferior Extensor Retinaculum

POSTERIOR TIBIAL NERVE

- Posterior Tibial Nerve
- Lateral Plantar Nerve
- Medial Plantar Nerve
- Nerve to Abductor Digiti Quinti Muscle
- Calcaneal Branches
- Heel Spur
- Abductor Hallucis Muscle

COMMON SITES OF NERVE ENTRAPMENT

behind the medial malleolus. In this passage the nerve faces the dangers of the posterior tibial artery and vein, the flexor hallucis longus, the posterior tibial, and were that not enough, the flexor digitorum longus tendons. This passage is called the tarsal tunnel, and it is rife with opportunities for entrapment.

Such entrapment, and the compression injuries it engenders, can result from direct trauma, ankle sprains, and ankle fractures. In such cases diagnosis is more or less straightforward. Greater diagnostic difficulty is encountered when the cause is less obvious: ganglionic cyst, lipoma, damage to an accessory bone called the os trigonum, or a stretching of the posterior tibial nerve resulting from extreme pronation.

Patients whose pain is an expression of these posterior tibial problems typically experience pain in the posterior medial ankle (directly below the tarsal tunnel), but often the symptom is medial or lateral plantar pain, heel pain, or pain in the medial longitudinal arch. On occasion there is even interdigital discomfort.

A positive Tinel's sign is often present and can be identified by the telltale tingling that follows tapping of the nerve in the tarsal tunnel with the neurological hammer. As is the case with saphenous problems, activity worsens the situation and magnifies the burning and tingling sensations, though these sensations are typically felt most strongly at night.

Certain diagnosis of posterior tibial problems requires electrodiagnostic tests that measure the time it takes an impulse to travel a known distance along the nerve.

Treatment usually consists of injection of anti-inflammatory medications to the area of entrapment, rectification of any arch problems that might be contributing to the entrapment by prescription of orthotics, and various physical therapies. On occasion such conservative treatments fail, and surgical decompression of the entrapped nerve is required.

Fitness walkers and, particularly, joggers and runners often complain of heel and foot pain that is traceable to pressure on the *calcaneal and plantar nerves,* which are branches of the posterior tibial nerve. The pain is often described as a dull, aching throb-bing at the medial or mid-plantar heel area. A sign that this is the issue is the reduction, often elimination, of pain when the foot is at rest and an increase when it is bearing weight. The pain is often exacerbated by a stretching injury to the mid-heel area from a plantar fasciitis exacerbated by ill-advised running or jumping.

One of the difficulties with neurological pain in the heel is the host of possible causes. In runners we often see heel pain resulting from pressure near the origin of the abductor muscle or at the point where the calcaneal and lateral branches of the posterior tibial nerve pass beneath the fascia layer. As a result the nerve becomes entrapped. Matters are made worse by additional pressure caused by stretching of the foot by running without proper prepa-ration, enlargement of the abductor hallucis muscles from overex-ercising, or trauma from a fall or a blow striking the heel.

Since the point of greatest pain usually overlies the area of en-trapment, orthotics are usually indicated here. Well-fitted orthotics correct the balance of the foot and remove the excess pres-sure causing the problem. Steroidal injections at the areas of great-est tenderness are also very effective.

Neuroma is a fairly common compressive neuropathy that is often referred to as neurofibroma, perineurofibrosis, neurinoma, and Morton's metatarsalgia.

Whatever the terminology, the case is an accumulation of col-lagenous material of the sheath of Schwann. This occurs only in the peripheral nerves, most commonly at the level of the third meta-tarsal interspace. Because such nerves receive branches from the medial and lateral plantar nerves, they are anatomically large to begin with. Growths can occur in many areas of the foot, but are most often found at the second and third metatarsal interspaces.

While extreme pronation is the usual culprit, tight and high-heeled shoes can also cause impalement. Such impingement and irritation to the nerve lead to a cycle of enlargement and swelling, ultimately forming an intraneural scar or neuroma, and of course the larger the nerve becomes, the easier it is to irritate.

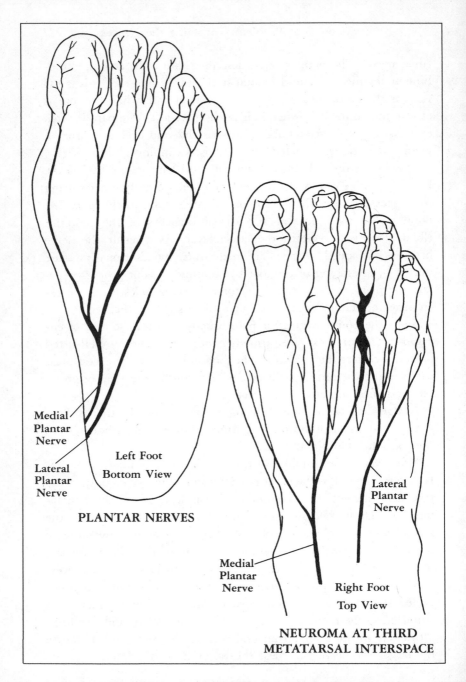

Medial
Plantar
Nerve

Lateral
Plantar
Nerve

Left Foot
Bottom View

PLANTAR NERVES

Lateral
Plantar
Nerve

Medial
Plantar
Nerve

Right Foot
Top View

**NEUROMA AT THIRD
METATARSAL INTERSPACE**

As was the case with posterior tibial and sural nerve injuries, pain primarily accompanies weight-bearing activities. Tingling, burning, numbness, and "pins and needles" are commonly associated with interdigital neuroma. Women suffer from this syndrome more than do men, an injustice probably owing to high-heeled shoes. While pain is usually experienced in only one of the feet, it can be extreme when the area between the second or third and fourth metatarsal heads is palpated. Night pain is uncommon.

Conservative therapeutic modalities often work, but occasionally surgery is called for.

Compartment syndromes occur more commonly in the lower extremity than in the upper extremity. There are four well-defined fascial compartments in the leg: the anterior, the peroneal, and two posterior tibial compartments. Muscles, nerves, and blood vessels pass through these fascial bound compartments.

When there is swelling of the muscular contents beyond the limits of the elasticity of the fascia, increased pressure on the enclosed muscles, blood vessels, and nerves result. It causes pain and can even impede blood flow, especially the venous return. Scarring can occur in the nerves and muscles.

These problems can occur in long-distance runners. If the cause of the swelling can be found and eliminated, such as running fewer miles, the condition will improve dramatically. Rarely is surgery required.

These syndromes are discussed in greater detail in the chapter on running.

Common Foot Problems
Involving the Bones

Most of the problems that bring patients to the foot doctor concern the soft areas of the foot. That is why so much of this book discusses corns, callouses, and the like. However it is problems of the bones of the foot that are generally the most serious faced by doctor and patient, and it is these we discuss in this chapter.

God did not give us feet so that we could be tickled or stabbed by tacks. We have feet because, as beings that walk upright, we need something to support us both statically (standing up) and dynamically (walking or running). The fact that the foot manages to do this at all is a miracle. (Try designing a steady, self-propelled 200-pound object capable of moving in any direction without giving it feet; even nature hasn't managed this at a macroscopic level.)

Nevertheless, the foot doesn't do this all that well, and that's why we have podiatrists. We stood upright a relatively short time ago, and nature hasn't had time to work out all the kinks. Thus there are a good number of forefoot and rearfoot bone problems that can be the cause and/or the effect of a disruption of the delicate biomechanical balance that has permitted us to roam the globe and to dust off the tops of refrigerators.

Flatfoot. Yup, this is just what you think it is. It's the same as fallen arches, and it's something you don't want.

It is important to understand that while "flat feet" describes a single condition, this condition can be the result of a number of separate causes. Moreover you can be born with flat feet or can get them as a result of traumatic injury or disease. While the congenital type of flat feet are the more common, many people born with this condition never suffer any symptoms. Either their genes compensate for the condition by giving their bodies a biomechanical leverage for which flat feet are no problem or their early life experience molds their bodies in such a way that their flat feet can handle the load.

But some people who are born with flat feet do have problems. Other people with congenitally flat feet have problems that could be helped but are not sufficiently debilitating (or are not known by them to be amenable to medical help) to bring the person suffering the minor problems to the doctor. For example, many people have flat feet that render their gait inefficient. As a result they tire easily when walking or find walking mildly painful, but think that this is the way it is for everyone. During World War II many potential inductees were rejected for having flat feet that would not have caused them any problems.

Many people, however, develop flat feet as a result of physical injury, rheumatoid arthritis, or one of a variety of neurological diseases. It is these people who usually become symptomatic. At one time there was little that could be done for people not willing to wear shoes that looked like two portable radios.

In recent years, however, the jogging boom has fueled the development of orthotics, supports that do for a patient what nature didn't. They can improve a whole range of undesirable foot conditions.

Unlike flat feet, *weak arches* nearly always cause problems. It is easy to tell if you have weak arches: They look normal when you

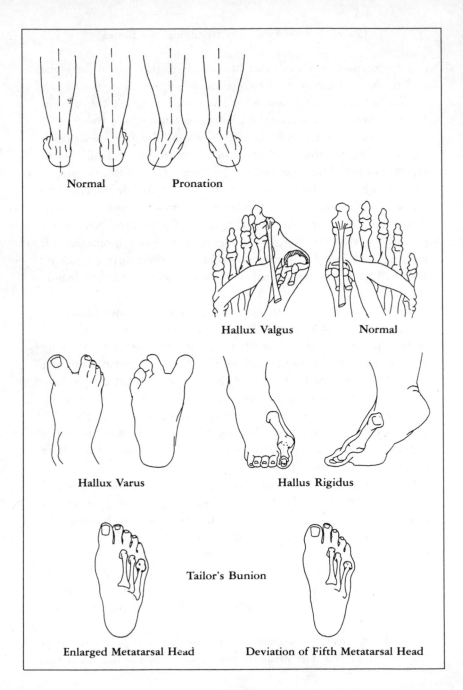

Normal   Pronation

Hallux Valgus   Normal

Hallux Varus   Hallus Rigidus

Tailor's Bunion

Enlarged Metatarsal Head   Deviation of Fifth Metatarsal Head

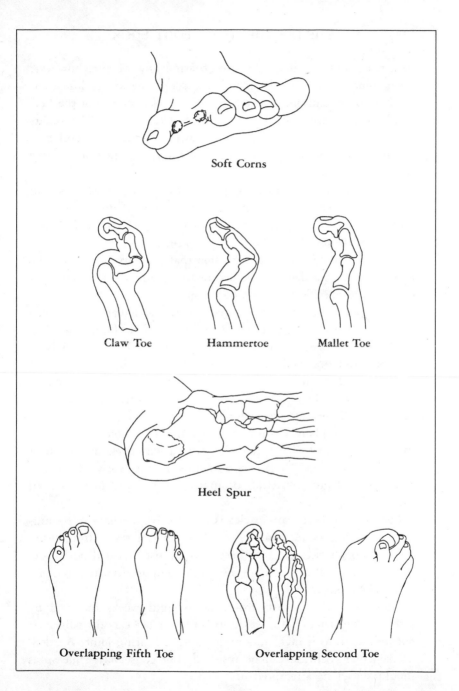

Soft Corns

Claw Toe   Hammertoe   Mallet Toe

Heel Spur

Overlapping Fifth Toe   Overlapping Second Toe

are sitting and the arches are not bearing any weight; however, when someone with weak arches stands up, the arches lose their contour and definition. Viewed from the back, the top of the heel will be seen to tilt inward, the collapse of the arch will be apparent, and the forefoot will pronate. However, it takes careful biochemical examination by a podiatrist to determine the exact degree of tilt and pronation.

A particularly pernicious aspect of weak-arch problems is that many of them concern areas of the foot far removed from the arch. Bunions, tailor's bunion, difficulties with metatarsals, and a host of other maladies all can have their origin at the arch.

Peroneal spastic flatfoot is a condition that presents as a rigid-type flatfoot. It is considered to be secondary to any subtalar joint pathology and specifically tarsal coalitions.

Tarsal coalitions are abnormalities of the articulations between the tarsal bones of the rearfoot. They can be of a fibrous nature, a cartilaginous bone, or an actual bony bridge. It seems to be a dominant inherited trait that occurs more commonly among males, with race playing no significant role. It is not a terribly common problem, but when it occurs, the preferred sites are the talocalcaneal and the calcaneonavicular areas.

Patients complain of stiffness and limited motion when trying to invert their foot. There can be localized tenderness directly over the site of coalition. These bars do not ossify until early adulthood, and the resulting restriction of motion is not pronounced until then.

Spasm of the peroneal muscles is a protective mechanism secondary to the loss of motion. Peroneal spasm can result from other inflammatory processes, and these causes must be ruled out before considering tarsal coalition. X rays and computerized tomography reveal their presence.

Short-leg walking casts from six to eight weeks followed by orthotics sometimes help. Resection of the talocalcaneal coalition is not indicated, as it involves a major weight-bearing joint. A calcaneonavicular coalition can be resected, but conservative measures should always be attempted first.

Pes cavus is the opposite of the weak arch. Pes cavus is the name foot people give to the high arch. Because a high arch is caused by muscle imbalance, and because such imbalances vary tremendously from person to person, the symptoms generated by high arches can be so different as to seem to come from different sources. Nonetheless the symptoms suffered by all these people can be relieved by treatment for the high arch that causes them. Because high arches alter the gait, they can cause pain in the legs as well as the feet. Among the more common symptoms of this problem are such forefoot lesions as callouses and hammertoes.

Conservative treatment of high arch can be as simple as a change of shoe and vigorous stretching exercises to keep the foot as supple as possible. More radical treatment includes various sources of surgery, such as cutting the plantar fascia or transferring tendons, the choice of which surgery being determined by the severity of the deformity. Such treatments are undertaken only if moderate techniques fail.

To this point we have examined rearfoot problems associated with arch height. Such problems are nearly always the forerunners of the forefoot problems that plague so much of the adult and elderly population. Now we shall examine some of the more common forefoot problems that also involve the bones of the feet.

A *bunion* is probably the most universally recognized of all foot problems. Because everyone has heard of bunions, most people are surprised to learn that those who actually have bunions usually don't know that they have them. Bunion victims, like all of us, tend to ignore problems until pain develops.

That, incidentally, is why we have pain. Perhaps in the long-ago, evolutionary past there may have been some other warning system, but it seems to be a part of what we are now that we ignore every warning except pain. Pain hurts (that's it's most notable property), and the hurt will succeed in getting us to the doctor where no other warning will.

So it is with the millions who develop bunions. Then they come to the doctor and learn that a bunion is a swelling at the inside portion of the first metatarsal head. It results in a deviation of the great toe in the direction of the outside of the foot. This deformation is called a *hallux valgus deformity* and it is about as unpleasant as its name implies. Hallux valgus can spread far beyond its source and is a familiar feature of a range of complex problems.

This problem is often congenital. But as is so often the case, even those spared the genes responsible for hallux valgus have developed a method for contracting the malady: modern fashionable footwear.

Not surprisingly, then, bunions more often victimize women than men. In many cases conservative management can alleviate the problem. Patient education, proper footwear, shoe padding, orthotics, localized physiotherapy, local injections of steroids, and other systemic medications to reduce swelling have all proven successful in relieving symptoms. In more serious cases, surgery may be required. The forms of therapy indicated by serious bunion deformation are as varied, and as case-specific, as are the nonsurgical techniques. Thus a great deal of presurgical planning is required if the surgery is to be successful.

Some procedures involve the soft tissue only; others involve both soft tissue and bone. Sometimes bone is removed, as in the reduction of the bunion deformity. Sometimes cuts are made in the bone, as in osteotomies of the forefoot and/or rearfoot along with this removal. Sometimes the outer sesamoid bone is removed entirely. Sometimes the joint is replaced partially or completely with artificial implants. The list goes on.

If you cross your legs while sitting on the floor tailor-fashion, and pretend to sew by hand, you'll feel a discomfort on the part of the foot called the fifth metatarsal head. If you do this day after day (as tailors did), you'll develop a painful bunion on that spot. Indeed this is about the only way you can get *tailor's bunion;* it is very rarely congenital. It is sometimes called a bunionette.

Once the soft tissue over the fifth metatarsal head becomes enlarged, a bursa often forms and becomes calcified.

In mild to moderate cases a broad-toed shoe and padding can help. Physiotherapy, injections, and medications can relieve the symptoms as well.

If conservative measures fail, a surgical procedure is performed whereby the bursa is excised and the underlying enlarged bone is reduced in size.

Hallux varus is a condition where there is a pronounced medial deflection of the great toe, just the opposite of hallux valgus. The congenital form is noticed shortly after birth. It usually responds well to conservative treatment.

The acquired type will follow unsuccessful hallux valgus surgery where the first toe is overcorrected. Further surgery is necessary to correct the problem.

Hallux extensus is a condition where the first toe is held in an extended or dorsiflexed position. It is also called *hallux elevatus.* It can occur after unsuccessful hallux valgus surgery and from rheumatoid arthritis. If painful, surgery is usually required.

If a doctor told you that you had *hallux rigidus,* he was saying the same thing as if he'd said you had *hallux limitus.* This is a problem of the first metatarsophalangeal joint. It is capable of impeding motion, slightly or completely, by locking the joint altogether. Usually an affliction of men, hallux rigidus can be either a primary affliction or a secondary result of hypertrophic arthritis, gout, or rheumatoid arthritis.

Hallux rigidus is usually discovered, or at least verified, by an X ray showing a narrowed joint surrounded by enlarged bone. Therapy always includes an increase in shoe size and stiffness. In severe cases conservative moves such as giving steroid injections and padding shoes rarely works. Sometimes removal of the joint is the only way to eliminate the pain, but often surgical removal of all the enlarged bone and placing an implant in the remaining part of the phalanx suffices to space the joint and alleviate the pain.

Metatarsalgia, which simply means pain in the metatarsal area, is a common source of foot discomfort. Women who wear extremely high-heeled shoes that overload the forefoot can attest to this. Crowding of the toes in a pointed-toe shoe can play a role. In plantar-flexed feet due to a short Achilles tendon, metatarsalgia is often present. High arches and abnormalities in metatarsal length can also lead to difficulties.

In the case of a short first metatarsal the work load not carried by it must be shifted to the lesser metatarsals. This can lead to a stress fracture of the second metatarsal, known as a march fracture, discussed in another chapter.

Treatment is conservative and directed first toward relief of pain. Nonsteroidal anti-inflammatories and commercially available metatarsal pads to relieve pressure can be helpful. Always be careful to place the pad in the area behind the metatarsal heads. A misplaced pad can lead to further difficulties. Orthotics help.

Manipulation and exercise of muscle tissue in the localized area can be very effective. Each metatarsophalangeal joint, from the first to the fifth, is grasped and put through its complete range of motion.

A variety of exercises designed to strengthen the muscles in the area can be performed. Trying to pick up a pencil or a golf ball or marble with the toes is effective. Grasping and pulling a towel with the toes is another common exercise.

The most common problem associated with the metatarsals is painful *callouses* that occur on the bottom of the foot. They have been described briefly in the chapter dealing with problems of the skin.

A painful callous can occur under any or all of the metatarsal heads, a weight-bearing surface. The callous can appear as a generalized thickened area of the skin or with a core or nucleated center. They can be very thick and the core very deep.

The condition is usually associated with a downward flexion of the metatarsal. In long-standing cases the metatarsal head can actually enlarge from the repeated trauma of weight bearing. Conservative treatment consists of reducing the painful thickened skin, pads applied to the foot or inside the shoe, and orthotics. Corn pads, pads with acid, and liquids with acid can be very dangerous and should be used only on the advice of a professional. Trimming one's own callouses can lead to serious infection.

If conservative treatment proves unsuccessful, there are a variety of surgical procedures available. Again, whenever you hear of lots of treatments, it usually tells you that there is no one ideal solution to the problem.

Underneath the head of the first metatarsal there are two normally occurring *sesamoid bones* that can come in all shapes and sizes. They can often appear to be fractured when they are not. They have been mentioned briefly in other chapters.

Because of their location they can be easily irritated by abnormalities in gait. When the normally well-distributed loads and forces incurred in gait are altered, the sesamoid bones can be subjected to repeated trauma with every step. This can lead to inflammation and callous formation. A plantar-flexed first metatarsal can add to the problem. These bones are also subject to routine traumatic injuries and can be the site of osteochondrosis in children. (See the chapter on the child's foot.)

Inflamed sesamoid bones occur frequently in athletes who are involved in high-impact sports and in dancers. They can be congenitally absent or extremely distorted or enlarged. On occasion they must be excised.

In addition to the two normally occurring sesamoid bones under the head of the first metatarsal there are many other frequently occurring *accessory bones* in the feet.

An *os trigonum* is a small bone that appears at the posterior process of the talus. It can cause pain in the retro-calcaneal space (behind the Achilles tendon).

Os tibiale externum, also called accessory navicular, occur at the medial aspect of the navicular bone. They can be quite large and cause considerable pain because of pressure from shoes.

Os peroneum in the tendon of the peroneus longus occur at the outside of the foot near the cuboid bone.

Others can occur almost anywhere in the foot, but the ones that appear under the great toe can cause a painful callous formation. Excision usually resolves the problem.

Overlapping toes is nearly always an inherited condition, and usually involves the fifth toe overlapping the fourth in both feet. Other toes are affected less frequently. It can also occur after unsuccessful joint surgery, but fortunately this is rare. If they are not a problem, which is often the case, they should be left alone. Surgery can usually resolve the problem. The earlier the treatment, the better the result.

Clubfoot, the technical name for which is talipes equinovarus, is a complicated congenital problem. The rearfoot is extremely plantar-flexed, with the forefoot going downward and inward. One out of every thousand newborn boys and twice as many girls have this condition.

Because the degree of deformity varies, the treatment can vary from the application of tape, soft castings, hard serial castings, and braces, to some very carefully planned, sophisticated surgery. Treatment must commence the minute the condition is recognized. This problem is discussed in the chapter on the child's foot as well.

Ever jump out of bed in the morning and have your foot literally go out from under you because of heel pain? You probably have a *heel spur,* known technically as inferior calcaneal spur syndrome.

Particularly likely to afflict males over forty, heel spurs are easily identifiable by X ray. Interestingly X ray will often expose spurs on both feet, whereas only one of these spurs will cause pain.

The first remedy to try is bathing the affected foot in warm (not hot) water and Epsom salts and, after drying, to carefully massage the feet with hand lotion. When such baths help but are not sufficient to eradicate pain, complementing the baths with pads, therapeutic nerve blocks, foam-rubber heels, and other conservative modalities will usually do the job. In all cases elevation of the feet whenever possible is highly recommended.

As is invariably the case with foot problems, some heel spurs are not amenable to conservative modalities. In such cases you guessed it, surgery is required. The primary surgical technique is the obvious one of making an incision in the side of the foot and removing the spur.

Some heel spurs are of a different sort. These, known as *Haglund's disease,* are usually referred to as pump bump. They attack the upper back of the heel. Therapy is the same as for other heel spurs, except that surgery, in the few cases that require it, consists of a reduction of the posterior superior aspect of the calcaneus.

Bone Tumors

First the good news: Primary bone tumors, even of the benign type, rarely develop in the foot. So it isn't necessary to buy life insurance the minute you see a lump on your foot; the odds are overwhelming that it's one of the non-life-threatening problems we have discussed.

The even better news is that, even when you have a tumor of the foot, it is in all likelihood benign. True, *benign* isn't the first word that springs to the mind of a person who has an *exostosis* under the nail. This tumor is very painful and often requires surgery. It is not malignant, however, and surgery virtually always solves the problem.

The best news is that many foot tumors are not only benign but asymptomatic. Unless a tumor, such as a *solitary bone cyst,* enlarges to the point that it fractures something in the area around it, you'll probably never know you have it.

An *enchondroma,* a cartilagineous lesion that is usually asymptomatic, acts in the same way.

A *fibroma* will sometimes occur in the heel bone, but, it, too, is usually asymptomatic.

The bad news is that there are some malignant tumors of the foot that we can do little about. If you are reading this, the odds are tremendously in your favor that you don't have such a tumor.

Osteosarcoma is a highly malignant tumor that fortunately occurs in the feet less than one percent of the time.

A *Ewing's sarcoma* is a malignant tumor of childhood that has the worst prognosis of any of the primary sarcomas of bone. Unfortunately it can occur in the foot about 5 percent of the time.

Chondrosarcoma is a slow-growing malignant tumor that occurs in middle-aged adults and involves the foot about one percent of the time. This tumor will usually metastasize to the lung.

There are several metabolic bone diseases that affect the foot.

Osteoporosis is a common disease and is often difficult to treat. It is a state of less bone being present than is normal for the person's age and sex. It occurs in the foot in the form of *Sudeck's atrophy,* which occurs most commonly in women who sustain a minor injury to the foot that causes them to overreact to their injury by not using the foot for a long period of time. Essentially the density of the bone is decreased and the bone porosity is increased.

Sufferers complain of severe burning pain and aching at the site of injury. The part is often warm and swollen.

Treatment is difficult. Reassuring the patient and relief of anxiety play an important role. Exercise, physiotherapy, analgesics, and massage can be helpful.

Osteomalacia differs from osteoporosis in that there is an increased loss of bone mineral compared with bone osteoid. The bone becomes more rigid. In children it's called rickets and is caused by a lack of vitamin D. It is rare today.

Finally, *gout* is an inherited disease seen mostly in older men; an increase in blood uric acid leads to deposits of uric acid crystals in the joints, most commonly the first metatarsophalangeal joint.

Rheumatoid arthritis, a chronic inflammatory disease of unknown cause, can involve the bones of the feet causing significant deformities. Any or all of the bones can be affected.

Claw toe, hallux valgus with bunion deformity, calcaneal spurs, and metatarsal involvement with painful callouses are common. Soft tissues can be involved also. Rheumatoid tendon nodules, if subjected to irritation, can be very painful. Conservative treatment consists of attention to localized painful lesions and often special molded shoes.

There is a juvenile form of the disease that occurs in children and adolescents under the age of sixteen. During childhood, treatment consists of local joint care. Flexion contracture of the toes, bunions, and rearfoot deformities are treated with the view to keep the joints as well aligned as possible. When adulthood is reached, the more severe deformities can be treated surgically.

Polyarthritis, associated with *psoriasis,* can cause nail and joint changes with a typical sausage-shaped swelling of the toes. It is a hereditary problem that often involves the hands and the feet. Treatment is conservative and surgery is rarely indicated.

All of these metabolic bone problems are discussed in greater detail in the chapter on the arthritic foot.

Köhler, Freiberg, and Sever are three doctors whose names have been given to various forms of *osteochondrosis.* This is thought to be an insufficiency of the blood supply (avascular necrosis) to the still-growing bone centers of children. It most often involves the hip, knee, or certain bones of the feet. When it involves the navicular bone, it is called Köhler's disease. When the growing center at the back of the heel bone is the focus, it's called Sever's disease; with the second metatarsal head, it's Freiberg's infraction. (An infraction is an incomplete fracture.)

The cause of these diseases is not yet fully understood, but diagnosis is not difficult: The usual signal is pain in the feet after exercise or on palpation. These problems are self-limiting, and therapy consists of conservative techniques to alleviate pain until the end of growth brings about complete recovery. These problems are discussed further in the chapter on children's feet. Treatment is usually conservative, consisting of limiting exercise, shoe paddings or orthotics, and physiotherapy. Fortunately these problems are all self-limiting and will resolve when the growing center of the involved bone, called the epiphyseal plate, stops growing.

Glossary

Abate—to lessen or decrease.

Abduction—the withdrawal of a part from the axis of the body.

Acquired—not congenital, but incurred or obtained after birth.

Adduction—the act of drawing toward a center or toward a median line.

Adipose—fat.

Aerobe—a microorganism that can live and grow in the presence of free oxygen.

Amputation—the surgical cutting off of a limb or other part.

Anaerobe—a microorganism that lives and grows only in the absence of molecular oxygen.

Anesthesia—loss of feeling or sensation.

Anesthetic—a drug that produces anesthesia.

Anhidrosis—an abnormal deficiency of sweat.

Ankylosis—abnormal immobility and consolidation of a joint.

Antalgic—relieving pain, as in an antalgic gait.

Anterior—situated in front of or in the forward part of.

Anteriorinferior—situated in front and below.

Anteroposterior—pertaining to forward and rear.

Anterosuperior—situated in front and above.

Anteversion—the forward tipping of a part, as in the pelvis.

Anti-inflammatory—suppressing inflammation.

Aperture—an opening, as in aperture pad.

Arch—a structure with a curved outline, as in longitudinal and transverse in the foot.

Artery—a vessel through which blood passes away from the heart to various parts of the body.

Arthritis—inflammation of a joint.

Arthropathy—any joint disease.

Atrophy—a wasting away or diminution in size of a part.

Avulsion—tearing away of a part, as in avulsion fracture at the base of the fifth metatarsal.

Axon—the central core of a nerve fiber, which forms its essential conducting part.

Baths, contrast—immersion of a part alternately in warm and cold water.

Benign—not malignant.

Bilateral—having two sides or pertaining to both sides.

Bipartite—having two parts or divisions, as in sesamoid bones.

Blister—a localized collection of fluid in the epidermis separating it from underlying parts.

Bunion—a swelling of the bursa mucosa of the ball of the great toe.

Bunionette—a bunionlike enlargement of the head and side of the fifth metatarsal.

Bursa—a sac cavity filled with viscid fluid and situated at places in the tissues subjected to friction.

Bursitis—inflammation of a bursa.

Calcaneus—the heel bone.

Calcification—the process by which organic tissue becomes hardened by a deposit of calcium salts.

Calf—the fleshy mass at the back of the leg below the knee.

Callosity—a circumscribed thickening of the skin due to friction.

Cancellous—spongy, latticelike bony tissue.

Capillary—minute vessels that connect the arterioles and the venules.

Capsule—an enveloping structure around a joint.

Cartilage, articular—a thin layer on the joint surfaces of bones.

Causalgia—a burning pain due to an injury to a peripheral nerve.

Cellulitis—a purulent inflammation of the loose subcutaneous tissue.

Chondritis—inflammation of cartilage.

Clubfoot—a congenitally deformed foot.

Condyle—a rounded projection on a bone.

Corn—a thickening of the skin produced by pressure and friction.

Coxa—the hip joint.

Cramp—a painful spasmodic muscular contraction.

Cuboid—a bone on the outer side of the tarsus, between the calcaneum and the fourth and fifth metatarsal bases.

Cuneiform—three wedge-shaped bones in the foot that articulate with the first, second, and third metatarsals anteriorly and the navicular bone posteriorly.

Cuticle—the epidermis, or outer layer of skin.

Cutis—skin.

Cyanosis—blueness of the skin.

Cyst—a sac that contains a semisolid substance.

Dactyl—a finger or toe.

Dactylitis—inflammation of a finger or toe.

Dactylomegaly—abnormally large size of fingers or toes.

Dead limb—the subjective sensation of numbness in a limb.

Deep—situated far beneath the surface.

Deformity—distortion of any part of the body.

Density—the quality of being compact.

Derm, derma—the skin.

Dermatitis—inflammation of the skin.

Desiccation—act of drying up.

Deviation—a turning away from the norm.

Digit—a finger or toe.

Digital—pertaining to a finger or toe.

Dipodia—duplication of a foot.

Disease—a definite morbid process having a characteristic train of symptoms.

Dislocation—the displacement of any part, especially bones.

Displacement—removal from the normal position.

Distal—remote; farther from any point of reference (as opposed to proximal).

Distally—in a distal direction.

Dorsal—the top of the foot.

Dorsiflexion—bending the top of the foot toward the front of the leg.

Dorsum—the top of the foot.

Dyshidrosis—any disorder of the perspiratory apparatus.

Eczema—inflammatory skin diseases with blisters, infiltration, water discharge, and the development of scales and crusts.

Edema—large amounts of fluid in the intercellular tissue spaces.

Epicondyle—an eminence upon a bone, above its condyle.

Epidermal—pertaining to the epidermis.

Epidermis—the outermost and nonvascular layer of the skin.

Epiphysis—growing center of cartilage in long bones.

Erosion—an eating or gnawing away.

Eruption—the act of breaking out.

Erythema—redness of the skin of many varieties.

Eversion—a turning outward.

Evert—to turn out.

Extension—a movement that brings the members of a limb into or toward a straight condition.

Extensor—any muscle that extends a joint.

Extrinsic—coming from or originating outside.

Fascia—a band of fibrous tissue that covers the body under the skin and invests the muscles and certain organs.

Fat—adipose tissue.

Fever—abnormally high bodily temperature.

Fibula—the outer and smaller of the two bones of the leg.

Fissure—any cleft or groove.

Flatfoot—a condition in which the medial longitudinal arch of the foot has flattened out.

Flex—to bend.

Flexion—the act of bending.

Flexor—any muscle that flexes a joint.

Foot—the terminal organ of the leg.

Fracture—a break in a bone.

Fungus—any one of a class of vegetable organisms of a low order of development.

Gait—the manner or style of walking. Antalgic gait—the avoidance of weight bearing on the affected side.

Ganglion—a cystic growth occurring on a tendon.

Gangrene—death or necrosis of tissue.

Genu—the knee.

Genu valgum—a deformity in which the knees are abnormally close together and the space between the ankles is increased (knock-knee).

Genu-varum—a deformity in which the knees are abnormally separated and the lower extremities are bowed inwardly (bowleg).

Hallucal—pertaining to the great toe.

Hallux—the great toe.

Hallux rigidus—painful flexion deformity of the great toe in which there is limitation of motion at the metatarsophalangeal joint.

Hallux valgus—displacement of the great toe toward the other toes.

Hallux varus—displacement of the great toe away from the other toes.

Heel—the hindmost part of the foot.

Hematoma—a tumor containing effused blood.

Hidrosis—the secretion and excretion of sweat.

Hypesthesia—excessive sensitivity of the skin.

Hyperhidrosis—excessive sweating.

Hyperkeratosis—hypertrophy of the corneous layer of the skin.

Hypertrophy—an enlargement of a part due to an increase in the size of its constituent cells.

Incision—the act of cutting.

Infection—invasion of the body by pathogenic microorganisms.

Intermittent—having periods of cessation of activity.

Interphalangeal—situated in a joint of a finger or toe between two phalanges.

Interspace—a space between two similar structures.

Intra—within.

Intrinsic —situated entirely within.

Inversion—a turning inward.

Invertor—a muscle that turns in a part.

Ischemia—local and temporary deficiency of blood, usually due to the contraction of a blood vessel.

Joint—the place of union or junction between two or more bones of the skeleton.

Keloid—a new growth or tumor of the skin.

Keratin—a protein that is the principal constituent of epidermis, hair, and nails.

Knee—the anterior aspect of the leg at the articulation of the femur and tibia.

Lateral—denoting a position more toward the side and father away from the medial plane.

Leg—the lower extremity between the knee and the ankle.

Lesion—any pathological discontinuity of tissue.

Leukonychia—a whitish discoloration of the nails.

Ligament—any tough, fibrous band that connects bones.

Limb—an arm or leg with its appendages.

Lipoid—fatlike.

Lipoma— a fatty tumor.

Maceration—the softening of tissues by soaking.

Malignant—virulent; tending to go from bad to worse.

Malleolus—a rounded process on either side of the ankle joint.

Marrow—the soft material that fills the cavities of the bones.

Mass—a body made up of cohering particles.

Massage—the systematic therapeutic friction, stroking, and kneading of the body.

Matrix, nail—the cells that grow the nail plate.

Medial—pertaining to the middle; nearer the median plane.

Melanin—the dark, amorphous pigment of the skin.

Melanoma, malignant—a tumor consisting of black masses of cells with a marked tendency to metastasis.

Membrane—a thin layer of tissue that covers a surface.

Metastasis—transfer of disease from one organ or part to another part not directly connected with it.

Metatarsal—a bone of the metatarsus.

Metatarsalgia—pain in the metatarsus.

Metatarsus—the part of the foot between the tarsus and the toes.

Muscle—an organ that by contraction produces the movements of an animal organism.

Mycosis—any disease caused by a fungus.

Nail—the horny dorsal plate on the distal phalanx of a finger or toe.

Navicular—a boat-shaped bone of the tarsus.

Necrosis—death of a cell or a group of cells that is in contact with living tissue.

Neoplasm—a new and abnormal growth.

Nerve—a cordlike structure that conveys impulses from one part of the body to another.

Neuralgia—paroxysmal pain that extends along the course of one or more nerves.

Neurilemma—the thin, membranous outer covering surrounding the myelin sheath of a nerve fiber.

Neurinoma—a specialized type of fibroma of nerves arising from the sheath of Schwann.

Neuritis—inflammation of a nerve.

Neuroma—a tumor growing from a nerve.

Neuropathy—a degenerative disease of a nerve or nerves.

Nevus—a circumscribed new growth of the skin of congenital origin that may be either vascular or nonvascular.

Numbness—a paresthesia of touch insensibility in a part.

Onychalgia—painful nails.

Onychatrophia—atrophy of a nail.

Onychauxis—overgrowth of the nails.

Onychia—inflammation of the matrix of the nail.

Onycho—combining form denoting relationship to the nails.

Onychocryptosis—ingrowing toenail.

Onychoelcosis—ulceration of the nail.

Onychogryptosis—a hooked nail.

Onycholysis—loosening or separation of a nail from its nail bed.

Onychomycosis—a disease of the nail caused by certain fungus organisms.

Onychopathy—disease of the nails.

Onychosis—deformity of a nail.

Os—bone.

Ossicle—a small bone.

Ossification—the formation of bone.

Osteitis—inflammation of a bone.

Osteoarthritis—chronic multiple degenerative joint disease.

Osteoarthropathy—any disease of the joints and bones.

Osteochronditis—inflammation of both bone and cartilage.

Osteochrondrosis—a disease of one or more of the growth centers in children.

Osteoma—a tumor composed of bone tissue.

Osteomalacia—softening of the bone.

Osteomyelitis—inflammation of bone caused by a pyogenic organism.

Osteophyte—a bony excrescence or osseous outgrowth.

Osteoporosis—abnormal porousness of bone.

Osteotomy—the surgical cutting of bone.

Palliative—affording relief, but not cure.

Pallor—paleness.

Palpation—the act of feeling with the hand.

Papule—a small circumscribed, solid elevation of the skin.

Parasite—a plant or animal that lives upon or within another living organism at whose expense it obtains some advantage without compensation.

Paresthesia—morbid or perverted sensation.

Patella—the kneecap.

Pathogen—any disease-producing organism.

Pedal—pertaining to the foot or feet.

Peri—a prefix meaning "around."

Perichondrium—the membrane that covers the surface of cartilage.

Periosteum—the tough, fibrous membrane surrounding bone.

Periostitis—inflammation of the periosteum.

Peripheral—situated at or near the periphery.

Periphery—the outward part or surface.

Pes—the foot.

Pes planus—a lowering of the medial longitudinal arch.

Pes pronatus—a deformed foot in which the outer border of the anterior part is higher than the inner border.

Pes supinatus—a deformed foot in which the inner border of the anterior part is higher than the outer border.

Phalanx—any bone of a finger or toe.

Plane—a flat surface determined by a position of three points in space.

Plantalgia—pain on the plantar surface of the foot.

Plantar—the sole of the foot.

Polyarthritis—an inflammation of several joints together.

Polyarticular—affecting many joints.

Porosity—the condition of being porous.

Prehallux—an extra bone of the foot found growing from the inner border of the navicular.

Prognosis—a forecast as to the probable result of an attack or disease.

Pronation—a combination of eversion and abduction in the rearfoot and forefoot that results in a lowering of the medial longitudinal arch.

Prophylaxis—the prevention of disease.

Proximal—nearest (opposite of distal).

Pruritis—intense itching.

Psoriasis—a skin disease of many varieties, characterized by the formation of scaly red patches on the extensor surfaces of the body.

Pus—a liquid inflammation product made up of cells and a thin liquid fluid called puris.

Pyogenic—producing pus.

Rash—a temporary eruption of the skin.

Reduction—the correction of a fracture.

Rehabilitation—the restoration of an injured patient to self-sufficiency.

Reinfection—a second infection by the same or similar agent.

Relapse—the return of a disease after its apparent cessation.

Resection—the excision of a considerable portion of an organ, especially the ends of bones and other structures forming a joint.

Retinaculum—a structure that retains tissue in its place.

Rheumatism—a disease marked by inflammation of the connective-tissue structures of the body, especially the muscles and joints.

Rigidity—stiffness or inflexibility.

Ringworm—a disease of the skin marked by the formation of ring-shaped pigmented patches covered with blisters.

Rotation—the process of turning around on axis.

Rubor—redness, one of the cardinal signs of inflammation.

Rupture—forcible tearing or breaking of a part.

Sac—a baglike structure.

Sagittal—an anteroposterior plane or section parallel to the long axis of the body.

Scale—a thin, platelike structure, as of epithelial cells compacted and shed from the skin.

Scaphoid—an older term for the navicular bone.

Sciatica—pain along the course of the sciatic nerve.

Sclerosis—hardening of a part from inflammation.

Sepsis—poisoning that is caused by products of a putrefactive process.

Septicemia—pathogenic bacteria and their associated poisons in the blood.

Sheath—a surrounding structure.

Shin—the anterior aspect of the leg below the knee.

Sign—any objective evidence of a disease.

Skeleton—the hard framework of the body.

Skin—the outer integument, or covering, of the body.

Sole—the bottom of the foot.

Spasm—a sudden involuntary contraction of muscle.

Splayfoot—flatfoot; talipes valgus.

Spur—a projecting piece of bone.

Stasis—a stopage of the flow of blood or other body fluid in any part.

Sudation—the process of sweating.

Sudor—sweat.

Superior—situated above.

Swelling—a transient abnormal enlargement or increase in volume of a body part.

Symptom—any functional evidence of disease.

Syndrome—a set of symptoms that occur together.

Synovia—a viscal fluid secreted by the synovial membrane contained in joint cavities, bursae, and tendon sheaths (synovial fluid).

Synovitis—inflammation of a synovial membrane.

System—the whole bodily organism.

Tabes—any wasting of the body.

Talipes—a congenital deformity.

Talus—the bone of the foot that articulates with the tibia and the fibula forming the ankle joint.

Tarsal—pertaining to the instep; any one of the bones of the rearfoot.

Tarsalgia—neuralgia of the foot.

Tarsus—the instep proper with its seven bones; the calcaneus, the talus, the navicular, the three cuneiforms, and the cuboid.

Tendinitis—inflammation of the tendons.

Tendo—tendon.

Tendon—the fibrous cord of connective tissue in which fibers of a muscle end and by which a muscle is attached to a bone.

Tensosynovitis—inflammation of a tendon sheath.

Thigh—the portion of the lower extremity that is situated between the hip above and the knees below.

Tibia—the inner and larger bone of the leg below the knee.

Tibialis—pertaining to the tibia.

Tinea—a fungus infection of the skin.

Toe—a digit of the foot.

Torsion—the act of twisting.

Toxin—any poisonous substance of microbic, vegetable, or animal origin.

Tuberosity—a broad eminence situated on a bone.

Tumor—a neoplasm; a mass of new tissue.

Ulcer—a loss of substance on a cutaneous or mucous surface, causing gradual disintegration and necrosis of the tissues.

Unction—an ointment.

Ungual—pertaining to the nails.

Unguis—a nail of a finger or toe.

Unilateral—affecting only one side.

Varico—combining form denoting twisted and swollen.

Varicose—unnaturally swollen vein.

Varicosity—a varicose vein.

Varus—bent inward.

Vaso—combining form denoting relationship to a vessel.

Vasodilator—any nerve or drug that causes dilation of the blood vessels.

Vein—a vessel that conveys the blood to or toward the heart.

Vena—a vein.

Verruca—a wart.

Vesicle—a small blister.

Virus—any living agent, submicroscopic.

Walk—to move on foot.

Walking—progressing on foot; the manner in which one moves on foot.

Wart—a localized benign hypertrophy of the skin, a verruca.

Wound—an injury to the body caused by physical means, with disruption of the normal continuity of body structures.

Zygodactyly—syndactyly, especially of the second or third fingers or toes.

The preceding glossary of terms was adapted from *Dorland's Illustrated Medical Dictionary,* 23rd ed., W. B. Saunders Company, 1957.

Useful Addresses

The following is a list of useful addresses. If for some reason a change occurs and the address that you find here is incorrect, telephone any local podiatrist; that person can give you the correct information.

The American Podiatric Medical Association
9312 Old Georgetown Road
Bethesda, MD 20814

Alabama Podiatric Medical Association
104–6 Lake Otis Medical Center
4050 Lake Otis Parkway
Anchorage, AL 99504

Arizona Podiatric Medical Association
5702 North 19th Avenue
Phoenix, AZ 85105

Arkansas Podiatric Medical Association
5517 John F. Kennedy Boulevard
North Little Rock, AR 72110

California Podiatric Medical Association
26 O'Farrell Street, #400
San Francisco, CA 94123

Colorado Podiatry Association
1380 Tulip Street, #C
Longmont, CO 80631

Connecticut Podiatric Medical Association
3446 Main Street
Stratford, CT 06497

DC Podiatric Medical Association
VA Medical Center
Montrose, NY 10548

Delaware Podiatric Medical Association
1701 Augustine Cutoff, #23
Wilmington, DE 19083

Federal Service Podiatric Medical Association
434 Westmark Avenue
Colorado Springs, CO 80906

Florida Podiatric Medical Association
410 North Gadsden Street
Tallahassee, FL 32301

Georgia Podiatric Medical Association
416 Broad Street SE
Gainesville, GA 30501

Hawaii Podiatric Medical Association
615 Piikoi Street, #1401
Honolulu, HI 96814

Idaho Podiatric Medical Association
203 12th Avenue
Nampa, ID 83651

Illinois Podiatric Medical Association
100 White Street
Frankfort, IL 60423

Indiana Podiatric Medical Association
201 North Illinois Street, #1910
Indianapolis, IN 46204

Iowa Podiatric Medical Society
5731 Urbandale Avenue
Des Moines, IA 50310

Kansas Podiatric Medical Association
615 South Topeka Boulevard
Topeka, KS 66603

Kentucky Podiatric Medical Association
3215 Dixie Highway
Erlanger, KY 41018

Louisiana Podiatric Medical Association
9830 Lake Forest Boulevard, # 117
New Orleans, LA 70127

Maine Podiatric Medical Association
1486 Broadway
South Portland, ME 04106

Maryland Podiatric Medical Association
1729 Glastonberry Road
Potomac, MD 20854

Massachusetts Podiatric Medical Society
14 Beacon Street, #804
Boston, MA 02108

Michigan Podiatric Medical Association
1003 North Washington Avenue
Lansing, MI 48906

Minnesota Podiatric Medical Association
825 Nicollet Avenue, #441
Minneapolis, MN 55402

Mississippi Podiatric Medical Association
1904 West Main Street
Tupelo, MS 38801

Missouri Podiatric Medical Association
PO Box 717
Jefferson City, MO 65102

Montana Podiatric Medical Association
907 South Main
Kalispell, MT 59901

Nebraska Podiatric Medical Association
7337 Dodge Street
Omaha, NE 68114

Nevada Podiatric Medical Association
2059 East Sahara, #D
Las Vegas, NV 89104

New Hampshire Podiatric Medical Association
168 Kinsley Street, #3
Nashua, NH 03061

New Jersey Podiatric Medical Society
Blason II, 505 South Lenola Road
Moorestown, NJ 08057

New Mexico Podiatric Medical Society
8008 Menaul Boulevard NE
Albuquerque, NM 87110

New York State Podiatric Medical Association
1255 Fifth Avenue
New York, NY 10029

North Carolina Podiatric Medical Society
PO Drawer 40399
Raleigh, NC 27629

North Dakota Podiatric Medical Association
1300 Gateway Drive
Fargo, ND 58103

Ohio Podiatric Medical Association
1490 Old West Henderson Road
Columbus, OH 43220

Oklahoma Podiatric Medical Association
P.O. Box 702225
Tulsa, OK 74170

Oregon Podiatric Medical Association
14495 Southwest Allen Boulevard, #101
Beaverton, OR 97005

Pennsylvania Podiatric Medical Association
757 Poplar Church Road
Camp Hill, PA 17011

Puerto Rico Podiatry Association
Cond San Martin, Pa23, #511
Santurce, PR 00909

Rhode Island Podiatry Society
1087 Warwick Avenue
Warwick, RI 02888

South Carolina Podiatric Medical Association
506 East Cheves Street, #202
Florence, SC 29506

South Dakota Podiatric Medical Association
808 South Minnesota Avenue
Sioux Falls, SD 57104

Tennessee Podiatric Medical Association
PO Box 50437
Nashville, TN 37205

Texas Podiatric Medical Association
5017 Bull Creed Road
Austin, TX 78731

Utah Podiatric Medical Association
144 South 700 East
Salt Lake City, UT 84102

Vermont Podiatric Medical Association
144 Woodstock Avenue
Rutland, VT 05701

Virginia Podiatric Medical Association
PO Box 1417, A-42
Alexandria, VA 22313

Washington State Podiatric Medical Association
PO Box 64255
Tacoma, WA 98464

West Virginia Podiatric Medical Association
55 15th Street
Wheeling, WV 26003

Wisconsin Society of Podiatric Medicine
2300 North Mayfair Road, #755
Wauwatosa, WI 53226

Wyoming Podiatric Medical Society
1471 Dewer Drive, #112
Rock Springs, WY 82901

Colleges of Podiatric Medicine

Barry University School of Podiatric Medicine
11300 Northeast Second Avenue
Miami Shores, FL 33161

California College of Podiatric Medicine
1210 Scott Street
San Francisco, CA 94115

College of Podiatric Medicine and Surgery
University of Osteopathic Medicine and Health Sciences
3200 Grande Avenue
Des Moines, IA 50312

Dr. William M. Scholl College of Podiatric Medicine
1001 North Dearborn Street
Chicago, IL 60610

New York College of Podiatric Medicine
53 East 124th Street
New York, NY 10035

Ohio College of Podiatric Medicine
10515 Carnegie Avenue
Cleveland, OH 44106

Pennsylvania College of Podiatric Medicine
Eighth at Race Street
Philadelphia, PA 19107

Selected References

Books

Altman, Morton I. *Modern Therapeutic Approaches to Foot Problems.* Mount Kisco, N.Y.: Futura Publishing Co. Inc., 1973.

American College of Foot Surgeons, *Complications in Foot Surgery.* Baltimore, The Williams & Wilkins Co., 1976.

Anthony, Catherine Parker. *Textbook of Anatomy and Physiology.* St. Louis: The C. V. Mosby Co., 1955.

Bateman, James E. *Foot Science.* Philadelphia: W. B. Saunders & Co., 1976.

Bateman, James E., and Arthur W. Trott. *The Foot and Ankle.* New York: Brian C. Decker, 1980.

Behrman, Richard E. *Pediatrics.* Philadelphia, W. B. Saunders & Co., 1987.

Berlin, Steven J. *Soft Somatic Tumors of the Foot: Diagnosis and Surgical Management.* Mount Kisco, N.Y.: Futura Publishing Co., Inc., 1976.

Brachman, Philip R. *Foot Therapy for Children.* Danville, Ill.: Interstate Printers and Publishers, 1966.

Brenner, Marc A. *Management of the Diabetic Foot.* Baltimore: Williams & Wilkins, 1987.

Calkins, Evan; Paul J. Davis, and B. Ford Amasa. *The Practice of Geriatrics.* Philadelphia: W. B. Saunders & Co., 1986.

Cecil, Russell, and Robert F. Loeb. *A Textbook of Medicine.* Philadelphia: W. B. Saunders & Co., 1959.

Conant, Norman F. *Manual of Clinical Mycology.* Philadelphia: W. B. Saunders & Co., 1959.

Coventry, Mark B. *The Year Book of Orthopedics and Traumatic Surgery.* Chicago: Year Book Medical Publishers, Inc., 1978.

Dobbs, Edward C. *Pharmacology and Oral Therapeutics.* St. Louis: The C. V. Mosby Co., 1956.

Dorland, W. A. Newman. *Medical Dictionary.* Philadelphia: W. B. Saunders, 1957.

Dubos, Rene J. *Bacterial and Mycotic Infections of Man.* Philadelphia: J. B. Lippincott Co., 1952.

Duvries, Henri L. *Surgery of the Foot.* St. Louis: The C. V. Mosby Co., 1959.

————. *Surgery of the Foot,* 4th edition. St. Louis: The C. V. Mosby Co., 1978.

Fielding, Morton D. *The Surgical Treatment of the Hallux-Abducto-Valgus and Allied Deformities.* Mount Kisco, N.Y.: Futura Publishing Co., Inc., 1973.

Gamble, Felton, and Irving Yale. *Clinical Foot Roengenology,* 2nd ed. Huntington Park, N.Y.: Robert E. Krieger Publishing Co., Inc.

Gannestras, Nicholas J. *Foot Disorders Medical and Surgical Management.* Philadelphia: Lea & Febiger, 1967.

Gray, H. *Anatomy of the Human Body,* 26th ed. Philadelphia: Lea & Febiger, 1956.

Hill, George J. *Outpatient Surgery*. Philadelphia: W. B. Saunders & Co., 1973.

Hlavac, Harry F. *The Foot Book, Advice for Athletes*. Mountain View, Calif.: World Publications, Inc., 1977.

Hunt, Gary C. *Physical Therapy of the Foot and Ankle*. New York: Churchill Livingstone, 1988.

Jahss, Melvin H. *Disorders of the Foot*, vols. I and II. Philadelphia: W. B. Saunders & Co., 1982.

Johanson, Donald, and Maitland Edey. *Lucy, The Beginnings of Humankind*. New York: Simon and Schuster, 1981.

Levin, Marvin E., and Lawrence W. O'Neal. *The Diabetic Foot*. St. Louis: The C. V. Mosby Co., 1977.

Lewi, Maurice. *Modern Foot Therapy*. Modern Foot Therapy Publishing Co., 1948.

Mann, Roger A. *Surgery of the Foot*. St. Louis: The C. V. Mosby Co., 1986.

Moeller, Fritz A. *The Surgical Treatment of Digital Deformities*. Mount Kisco, N.Y.: Futura Publishing Co., 1975.

Tobias, Norman. *Essentials of Dermatology*. Philadelphia: J. B. Lippincott Co., 1948.

Yale, Irving. *Podiatric Medicine*. Baltimore: The Williams & Wilkins Co., 1974.

Periodicals

Burns, Albert E., ed. "Digital Surgery," *Clinics in Pediatric Medicine and Surgery* 3, no. 1 (1986): 1–216.

Cagiulosi, Charles P., ed. "Minimal Incision Surgery," *Clinics in Podiatry* 2, no. 3 (1985): 413–585.

Delauro, Thomas M., and Rock G. Positanu, eds. "Occupational

Medicine," *Clinics in Podiatric Medicine and Surgery* 4, no. 3 (1987): 523–760.

Dockery, Gary L., ed. "Dermatology of the Lower Extremities," *Clinics in Podiatric Medicine and Surgery* 3, no. 3 (1986): 385–593.

Eickhoff, Renate. "Origin of Bipedalism—When, Why, How, and Where?" *South African Journal of Science* 84 (June 1988): 486–488.

Frykberg, Robert F., ed. "Emerging Technologies in Podiatric Medicine," *Clinics in Podiatric Medicine and Surgery* 4, no. 4 (1987): 767–1006.

Ganley, James V., ed. "Podopediatrics," *Clinics in Podiatry* 1, no. 3 (1984): 445–746.

Gordon, Gary M., and Jonathan P. Contompasis, eds. "Sports Medicine," *Clinics in Podiatric Medicine and Surgery* 3, no. 4 (1986): 595–791.

Grumbine, Nicholas, ed. "Plastic Surgery," *Clinics in Podiatric Medicine and Surgery* 3, no. 2 (1986): 221–383.

Harkless, Lawrence B., and Dennis Kenrick J. "The Diabetic Foot," *Clinics in Podiatric Medicine and Surgery* 4, no. 2 (1987): 315–522.

Helfand, Arthur E., and Bruno, Joseph, eds. "Rehabilitation of the Foot," *Clinics in Podiatry* 1, no. 2 (1984): 249–444.

Jules, Kevin T., ed. "Hallux Valgus and Allied Deformities," *Clinics in Podiatric Medicine and Surgery* 6, no. 1 (1989): 1–213.

Karlin, Jeffery M., ed. "Pediatric Surgery of the Foot and Ankle," *Clinics in Podiatric Medicine and Surgery* 4, no. 1 (1987): 1–313.

LaParta, Guido, ed. "Osteosynthesis in Foot and Ankle Surgery," *Clinics in Podiatry* 2, no. 1 (1985): 1–195.

Leuy, Leonard A., ed. "Systemic Diseases Affecting the Foot," *Clinics in Podiatry,* 2, no. 4 (1985): 591–791.

Oloff, Lawrence M., ed. "Rheumatology," *Clinics in Podiatric Medicine and Surgery* 5, no. 1 (1988): 1–257.

Oloff-Solomon, Joan, ed. "Radiology of the Foot and Ankle," *Clinics in Podiatric Medicine and Surgery* 5, no. 4 (1988): 759–985.

Rzonca, Edward C.; Thomas Delauro; and Rock Positano, eds. "Applied Biomechanics," *Clinics in Podiatric Medicine and Surgery* 5, no. 3 (1988): 443–758.

Schnabel, Truman G.: "The Dangers of Dress: Medical Hazards in Fashion and Fads," *Transactions of the American Clinical and Climatological Association* 97 (1985): 183–190.

Scurran, Barry L., ed. "Osseous Trauma of the Foot," *Clinics in Podiatry* 2, no. 2 (1985): 199–410.

———. "Selected Topics in Medicine and Surgery," *Clinics in Podiatric Medicine and Surgery* 5, no. 2 (1988): 267–442.

Weil, Lowell Scott, ed. "Implants in Foot Surgery," *Clinics in Podiatry* 1, no. 1 (1984): 1–245.

Clinics in Podiatry and *Clinics in Podiatric Medicine and Surgery* are published by W. B. Saunders & Co., Philadelphia.

Countless issues of the following publications were consulted:

Journal of American Podiatric Medical Association
Arthritis Information Magazine
Consultant
Emergency Medicine
Journal of Foot Surgery
Geriatrics
Journal of Musculoskeletal Medicine
The Physician and Sports Medicine
Practical Cardiology

Correspondence

Extremely helpful information was obtained via correspondence with the following:

The American Podiatric Medical Association
9312 Old Georgetown Road
Bethesda, MD 20814

American Sporting Goods Corporation
16542 Milliken Avenue
Irvine, CA 91714

Brooks Shoes Inc.
9341 Courtland Drive
Rockford, MI 49351

Drew Shoe Corp.
252 Quarry Road
Lancaster, Ohio 43130

Jerry Miller, I.D. Shoes
Marble Street
Whitman, MA 02383

Reebok International Ltd.
150 Royall Street
Canton, MA 02021

INDEX